The COTA in the Schools

Tracie Barlow, OTR/L

Joanne Pinkava, OTR/L

Laurie L. Gombash, M.Ed., PT

**Therapy
Skill Builders®**
a division of
The Psychological Corporation
555 Academic Court
San Antonio, Texas 78204-2498
1-800-228-0752

D1154030

To our co-workers and students,

especially Shelly, Kathy, and Jean,

for their encouragement and support

About the Authors

Tracie Barlow, OTR/L, is a pediatric occupational therapist working in a public preschool setting in Northwest Ohio. She is certified in the Neuro-Developmental Treatment (NDT) approach and specializes in the treatment of infants and children with neurological impairments. Tracie has worked in a variety of pediatric facilities, including hospital-based settings, private practice, outpatient clinic, early intervention programs, and school-based settings. She has been active in the clinical education of both COTA- and OTR-level students. She also has been a clinical lecturer at several local colleges. Tracie earned her Bachelor of Science degree in Occupational Therapy from Mount Mary College in Milwaukee, Wisconsin in 1989. She lives near Liberty Center, Ohio with her husband Robb and their two-year-old daughter Erica.

Joanne Pinkava, OTR/L, graduated from Ohio State University in 1973 with a Bachelor of Science degree in Occupational Therapy. She has worked in the public schools for twenty years in urban and rural settings and is active in the education of OTR students. She lives with her husband, four children, and their three dogs.

Laurie L. Gombash received a Bachelor of Science degree in Physical Therapy from the Medical College of Ohio in Consortium with Bowling Green State University and the University of Toledo. She developed an interest in vestibular rehabilitation and co-authored several articles on vestibular rehabilitation and treatment before deciding on a career in the pediatric field. For the past four years, Laurie has worked as an early intervention physical therapist and a school-based physical therapist in rural northwestern Ohio. In 1997, she received her Master of Education degree at the University of Toledo and an early intervention certificate. She has served as Executive Board Member of the Medical College of Ohio Alumni Association and Clinical Lecturer at the Medical College of Ohio Hospitals. Laurie has been very involved with clinical education and has served as a clinical instructor for numerous physical therapy students and physical therapist assistant students over the past fourteen years. She lives on an 80-acre farm with her husband and their three children.

Contents

Preface

THIS MANUAL IS WRITTEN to assist the certified occupational therapy assistant (COTA) who is working in the school system. COTA students, entry-level COTAs, or COTAs with little or no school-based experience can use the information. This manual is not intended to offer the knowledge or to present the skills needed for advanced or specialty practice in pediatric occupational therapy.

The manual is organized into four chapters. Chapter 1 includes information on normal motor control, the developmental sequence, the influences of reflexes, and frames of reference in pediatric occupational therapy. Chapter 2 discusses school-based issues—the Multifactored Evaluation, the Individualized Education Plan, integrated therapy, and the role of the COTA in the school setting. Chapter 3 is a quick reference to many pediatric disorders seen in the school setting. Chapter 4 is full of therapy ideas and suggestions. Feeding, sensory-motor treatment, and a list of specialized equipment often used by school-based COTAs are highlighted.

Chapter 1

Normal
Motor Development

THE DEVELOPMENT OF NORMAL MOVEMENT is a continuing and dynamic process. Each child has an individual schedule for development that must be recognized and respected (Tecklin, 1989).

Motor control is the study of the nature and cause of movement. It encompasses both the control of posture and balance and the movement of the body in space. Competent pediatric therapists and assistants need an in-depth understanding and appreciation of normal motor development. Normal motor development must be the reference point that one uses to understand abnormal motor development and to implement effective treatment techniques. Although each child has his own time schedule for the development of motor skills, the maturation of the central nervous system (CNS) proceeds in a predictable sequence. One of the most important concepts about movement is that motor skill development is sequential.

Patterns of Growth and Development

1. The first directional concept of development is that it progresses cephalo-caudally—that is, from the head to the foot. An infant first gains voluntary head control before she gains lower extremity control for walking.

2. The second concept of directional development is that it occurs from proximal to distal. An infant bats at toys before he demonstrates the fine-motor skill of picking up an object.

3. The third concept of directional development is the reflex-to-voluntary movement. Initially, the neonate's movement patterns are dominated by reflexes, such as the asymmetrical tonic neck reflex, which is present when the infant's arm and leg on the face side extends and the arm and leg on the skull side flex. As these reflexes are integrated, more voluntary movements emerge without the influence of the reflex.

4. The fourth directional concept involves the direction of overall change in movement skill acquisition, which is from gross, large muscles to fine, more discrete movements. Initially, a toddler scribbles on paper before he starts coloring within the lines.

5. The last directional concept is that stability progresses into controlled mobility. A toddler is able to stand and gain stability in an upright position before she walks and becomes mobile.

Motor Milestones

GROSS-MOTOR MILESTONES

3 months	Prone, raises head 45 degrees to 90 degrees Prone on forearms
5 months	Rolls prone to supine Prone on extended arms
6 months	Sits independently propped on arms Rolls supine to prone
7–8 months	Commando crawls Pivot prone
8 months	Sits with arms free
8–9 months	Pulls to stand
9 months	Creeps Bear walks
9–10 months	Cruises
10–15 months	Walks
11–20 months	Walks backward
24 months	Jumps off floor, both feet

FINE-MOTOR MILESTONES

Newborn	Palmar grasp reflex
1–3 months	Swats at objects
3–4 months	Ulnar-palmar grasp (no thumb)
4–5 months	Palmar squeeze grasp (no thumb) Direct reach Hands to midline
5–6 months	Radial-palmar grasp
7–9 months	Transfers objects
7 months	Inferior scissors grasp (thumb abducted, opposes first two fingers to grasp a 1" cube)
8 months	scissor grasp
9 months	Inferior pincer grasp
10 months	Voluntary release begins Poking—index isolation Uses pincer grasp
11–12 months	Smooth release—large items Push release—small items
12 months	Fine pincer grasp
12–18 months	Palmar-supinate grasp
18 months	Precise grasp (prehension) Voluntary release Placement
2–3 years	Digital-pronate grasp
3½–4 years	Static tripod
4½–6 years	Dynamic tripod
5–6 years	Established hand dominance

DEVELOPMENTAL SEQUENCE

Prone

Flexion predominates	Newborn
Head—rotates side to side (pivot prone)	
Scapula—elevated and abducted	
Pelvis—posterior pelvic tilt	
Prone on elbows	1–2 months
Head—extends to 45 degrees, head more in midline	
Scapula—elevated, abduction to adduction	
Pelvis—decreased posterior pelvic tilt	
Prone on elbows	3–4 months
Head—extends to 90 degrees	
Scapula—elevated and abducted, depressed and adducted	
Pelvis—anterior tilt with extension	
Prone to supine	4–5 months
Prone on extended arms	5–6 months
Head—complete refinement	
Scapula—neutral, arms able to reach	
Pelvis—anterior tilt	
Commando crawls (belly crawl)	5–6 months
Assumes quadruped or four-point	5–6 months
Maintains quadruped	5–9 months
Rocks in quadruped	5–9 months
Reaches in quadruped	5–9 months
Creeping	7–9 months

Supine

Flexion with averted head	Newborn
Head—head lag with pull to sit	
Scapula—elevated	

Pelvic—posterior tilt

Sitting with support   1–2 months

Head—bobs, decreasing head lag

Scapula—decreased elevation, increased adduction

Pelvis—posterior tilt

Sitting with support   3–4 months

Head—steady and midline, increased anterior/posterior control

Scapula—hands to midline with abduction

Pelvis—neutral (abdominal)

Rolling supine to side   3–4 months

Head—flexes against gravity

Scapula—hands to midline with abduction

Pelvis—lower extremities off floor (abdominal)

Rolling supine to prone   5–6 months

Tripod sitting, reaching   5–6 months

Independent sitting, upper extremity play   7–9 months

Transitions sitting to prone and sitting   7–9 months
to four-point

Upright

Standing reaction/Automatic stepping	Newborn
Stands rigid pillar/Positive and negative support	4–5 months
Stands with wide base of support, supported	6–8 months
Bounces while standing with support	7–9 months
Kneels with hip flexion to hip extension	7–9 months
Heel sit to tall kneel to pull to stand	7–9 months
Stands and leans against support	7–9 months
Cruises sideways, turns	10–12 months
Stands with one hand held	10–12 months
Walks with two hands held	10–12 months
Stands independently	10–12 months

Upright *(continued)*

Stoops and recovers	10–12 months
(child bends down and stands up without hand support)	
Walks independently	13–15 months

STAGES OF ORAL-MOTOR DEVELOPMENT*

Age	Oral-motor pattern	Feeding skill
32–34 weeks Gestation	**Suck/swallow** Swallow initiated after suckle Tongue movement but not coordinated with respiration	Nonnutritive suckle Pacifier or finger
At term	**Suckle** Extension/retraction movement of tongue combined with up-down movements of mandible and coordinated with respiration	Nipple feeding
3–6 months	**Sucking** Up-down motion of tongue independent of graded jaw excursions	Spoon feeding of pureed foods
6–9 months	**Munching** Flattening and spreading of tongue with lateral move- ment for collection; finely graded and repetitive vertical jaw movements	Advance to small pieces of soft solids and soft finger foods
9–36 months	**Chewing** More controlled tongue lateralization patterns; rotary jaw movements to grind food	Advance to larger pieces of soft solids and more fibrous textures

*Source: Eicher 1998

ACTIVITIES OF DAILY LIVING (ADL) MILESTONES

6 months	Holds own bottle
9 months	Independently finger feeds
1 year	Pushes arms through sleeves and legs through pants
2 years	Holds and drinks independently from a small glass with one or two hands Drinks from a straw Removes unfastened coat Pulls off socks Takes off shoes if untied
2½ years	Puts on own coat (not including fasteners) Removes pull-down pants
2½ years	Feeds self independently with spoon with minimal spillage
3 years	Puts on shoes without fastening Unbuttons large front buttons
3½ years	Puts on pants independently Unzips front zipper on jacket Washes and dries face Toilet trained
4 years	Feeds self independently with fork Dresses and undresses with supervision (puts on pants, shirt, socks, shoes) Zips engaging zipper Brushes teeth
4½ years	Buttons, snaps, and zips independently Uses bathroom independently
5 years	Dresses and undresses unsupervised
6 years	Ties shoelaces independently
6–7 years	Uses a knife at mealtime

Reflexes

Reflexes play a critical role in the development of the child's movement abilities from birth. Reflexes are thought to provide the means by which a baby can interact with the environment and move against gravity at a time when controlled antigravity movement is otherwise limited (Tecklin, 1989). The spontaneous movements produced by reflex activity are important for later motor development.

Reflexes can be categorized as primitive or postural (Scherzer & Tscharnuter, 1982). Primitive reflexes are patterns of movement that are normally observed in the early stages of development. They are present at birth and are generally integrated by six months of age. When early reflexes persist longer than normal and interfere with normal developmental sequences, they are considered pathologic reflexes. Postural reflexes are high-level responses that assist the child in regaining and maintaining the body and head in an upright position. Righting and equilibrium reactions are examples of postural reflex reactions. Righting reactions develop between one and six months postnatally. With experience and maturation of the central nervous system, righting reactions integrate with equilibrium reactions and continue to function in automatic posture control and movement control for life. Equilibrium reactions function to maintain and regain balance during movement. Equilibrium reactions are the highest level responses that allow humans to function on two legs and to use the hands for manipulation while standing and moving (Tecklin, 1989).

As a baby develops and gains greater control of movement against gravity, the primitive reflexes decrease as the postural reactions appear. Postural reactions play an important role in the regulation and distribution of tone (Bobath, 1966). Normal tone has been described as the state of muscle tone that is high enough to permit movement against gravity, yet low enough to allow complete freedom of movement. A normal level of postural tone allows for ease of movement against gravity.

Primitive Reflexes

1. **Rooting**—Rooting helps the infant locate the food source. To stimulate, use a finger to lightly stroke the perioral skin at the corner of the infant's mouth. The infant responds by turning the face and tongue to the site of stimulation and activating sucking. The response is usually seen between birth and two months. Abnormal persistence of this reflex could interfere with oral-motor development, development of midline control of the head, and visual tracking.

2. **Moro**—Stimulate by holding the infant in a semi-seated position (support the head in midline with one hand and the back with the other hand). Allow the infant's head to drop backward a few inches. This should elicit a startle response (abduction and upward movement of the arms at the shoulders, with extension of the elbows and fingers as the hands open). The startle response is followed by adduction and flexion of the upper extremities and movement toward midline. The reflex is strongest at two months and is usually inhibited by four to six months. Abnormal persistence of this reflex could interfere with balance reactions in sitting, protective responses in sitting, eye-hand coordination, and visual tracking.

3. **Palmar Grasp**—Stimulate by inserting a finger into the infant's hand from the ulnar side and press against the palmar surface to elicit the palmar grasp. The desired response from the infant is strong flexion of the fingers around the examiner's finger. The duration of the response is up to two to four months of age. Abnormal persistence of this reflex could interfere with the ability to grasp and release objects voluntarily and to weight bear on an open hand.

4. **Plantar Grasp**—Stimulate by applying pressure to the sole of the foot. The infant responds with strong flexion of the toes. Plantar grasp is integrated by twelve months, and becomes inhibited by weight bearing through the feet in standing. Abnormal persistence of this reflex could interfere with standing with feet flat, balance reactions and weight shifting in standing.

5. **Primary Standing Reflex** (Positive Support Reflex)—Stimulate by suspending the infant vertically with the trunk supported under the arms. The soles of the feet are brought into contact with a hard surface. The infant's reflexive response is to bear some weight through the feet. This reflex is present at birth and gradually disappears by two months of age. Abnormal persistence of this reflex

could interfere with standing and walking and weight shifting in standing. Also, it could lead to contractures of the ankles into plantar flexion.

6. **Primary Walking Response (Stepping Reflex)**—To stimulate, support the infant under the arms and hold upright with the trunk inclined slightly forward, which results in an alternating heel-toe gait pattern. This is strongest in the first few weeks of life and gradually disappears by two months of age. Abnormal persistence of this reflex could interfere with standing and walking, weight shifting in standing, and development of smooth and coordinated reciprocal movements of the lower extremities.

7. **ATNR (Asymmetrical tonic neck reflex)**—Stimulate by placing the infant in supine with the head in midline. Rotate the head 90 degrees and hold for five seconds. The reflex is present when the arm and leg on the face side extends and the arm and leg on the skull side flex. The response is more pronounced in the arms. The ATNR is seen most strongly in infants from birth to two months of age and is integrated by four to six months. Abnormal persistence of this reflex could interfere with feeding, visual tracking, midline use of the hands, rolling, bilateral hand use, and the development of crawling. Long-term negative effects include possible skeletal deformities such as scoliosis, hip subluxation, and hip dislocation.

8. **STNR (Symmetrical tonic neck reflex)**—To stimulate, hold the child in prone, and flex and extend the head. When the head is in flexion, arms are flexed and legs are extended. When the head is in extension, arms are extended and legs are flexed. The STNR is typically seen at four to six months and integrated by eight to twelve months. Abnormal persistence of this reflex could interfere with the ability to prop on arms in prone position, reciprocal crawling, and attaining and maintaining quadruped.

9. **Landau**—Stimulate by suspending the infant in prone with support under the trunk between the shoulders and pelvis. The infant responds with extension of the back and later of the hips and legs. This begins at four months and is mature by twelve to twenty-four months. Abnormal persistence of this reflex could interfere with prone propping and crawling.

10. **TLR (Tonic labyrinthine reflex)**—Stimulate this reflex by placing the infant in either prone or supine. The infant responds with generalized flexion when in prone and generalized extension when in

supine. This begins in the first month and is integrated by six to twelve months. Abnormal persistence of this reflex could interfere with rolling and the ability to transition into sitting from supine. Often it causes full body extension, which interferes with balance in sitting or standing.

Postural Reflexes

1. **Righting Reactions**—Serve to orient the head in space (upright) and in relation to the ground and to orient the head and body when rotation occurs. They often begin in the first month and reach full maturation by ten to twelve months.

   a. Body righting on the head reaction (BOH)—rights the head in response to the body touching the support surface.

   b. Optical righting—rights the head in relation to visual stimulation.

   c. Labyrinthine righting—rights the head and body in relation to vestibular stimulation caused by movement.

   d. Neck righting on body reaction (NOB)—with lateral displacement, the head attempts to right with continuation through the trunk to contribute to rolling.

   e. Body righting on body reaction (BOB)—allows the trunk to remain aligned during sequential rotation.

2. **Protective Reactions**—Sometimes known as parachute reactions. Extension of the extremities is seen as the body is moved downward, forward, sideways, and/or backward. Appears at seven to eight months and persists throughout life.

3. **Tilt/Equilibrium Reactions**—Automatic responses of the body and extremities used to sustain control either on an unstable base of support, where the supporting surfaces move under the body, or as the body moves over a stable base of support. Appears at seven to eight months and persists throughout life.

Frames of Reference in Pediatric Occupational Therapy

Occupational therapists and occupational therapy assistants use a frame of reference or theory to help organize and put into practice complex observations and behaviors of the children they see. The frame of reference assists a therapist in developing a child's individualized treatment plan and goals based on one or more specific theories. The therapist's frame of reference is the linkage between theory and practice (Hinojosa, Kramer, & Pratt, 1996).

There are many frames of reference used in pediatric occupational therapy, and no single theory can explain it all. In the next section, we will briefly outline some of the major frames of reference used in pediatric occupational therapy.

Spatiotemporal Adaptation

The spatiotemporal-adaptation frame of reference was proposed by Gilfoyle, Grady, and Moore in 1990 (Hinojosa, Kramer, & Pratt, 1996). Spatiotemporal adaptation is a continuous act of adjusting body processes required to function within a given space and time. Development is viewed as a spiraling process, moving from simplex to complex, where movement and more intricate patterns of adaptation evolve from more primitive behaviors. This process includes four major components: assimilation, accommodation, association, and differentiation. A key concept in this theory is that the maturation of the nervous system results from sensory input, motor output, and feedback. Another key idea is that sensory feedback from new experiences facilitates higher levels of adaptations.

Using this model, the COTA assists the child in modifying older, more primitive behaviors for effective motor responses rather than continually acquiring new skills.

The Developmental Frame of Reference

Lela Llorens, an occupational therapist, identified the developmental frame of reference (Hinojosa, Kramer, & Pratt, 1996), which focuses on the physical, social, and psychological aspects of life tasks and relationships. The COTA looks at individual functions and their integration during specific periods of life (horizontal development) as well as over the course of time (longitudinal development). The integration of these two aspects of life is essential for normal development.

Using this theory, the COTA acts as a change agent, facilitating the growth and development of a child.

Sensory Integration (SI)

The sensory-integration frame of reference was developed by A. Jean Ayres. This theory gives a broad developmental perspective on how the brain develops the capacity to perceive, learn, and organize behavior. Sensory integration is the process of organizing sensory input in the brain for the emitting of an adaptive response (Ayres, 1972). An adaptive response occurs when a child successfully meets an environmental challenge. The goal is to control sensory input to activate brain mechanisms. An adaptive response is encouraged to promote a purposeful and goal-directed activity following sensory stimulation. This activity should be fun, and the child should be actively involved. For example, it is not enough for a child to ride passively while spinning in a net swing; the child should be actively involved in playing a ring-toss game while swinging in the prone position.

There are a variety of sensory processing disorders such as tactile defensiveness, an underreactive vestibular system, an overreactive vestibular system, and dyspraxia (difficulty with movement and motor planning) that could benefit from SI treatment. The sensory systems that are important in the sensory integration theory include the auditory, visual, olfactory, tactile, vestibular, and proprioceptive.

Neurodevelopmental Treatment (NDT)

The neurodevelopmental-treatment frame of reference is based on the clinical experiences and personal views of Berta Bobath, a physiotherapist, and her physician husband, Karel Bobath. This theory is based on normal and abnormal development and reflects both sensory and motor development. The goal of this treatment approach is to inhibit abnormal movement patterns and facilitate normal movement patterns. The aim of NDT is to obtain changes in postural tone and patterns toward the more normal (Bobath, 1966). The importance of normalizing sensation also is an important component. Key points of control are used to influence a child's movement and regulate tone. NDT involves handling the child and providing graded sensory input to influence the motor output. Treatment is used for those children with sensory-motor dysfunction. It is a common approach used with the diagnosis of cerebral palsy. The theory incorporates treatment of the whole child. The approach is hands-on and the child is an active participant in the treatment session. The end goal of NDT is to improve sensory and motor skills to promote improved functional abilities.

Occupational Behavior

The occupational-behavior frame of reference first was developed by Mary Reilly. She defined occupational behavior as the use of day-to-day behaviors of daily living, including self-care, work, and play, to restore performance throughout the life span. In pediatrics, she focused on the importance of play in development. She saw play as having an organizing effect on a child's behavior. The theory emphasizes the importance of the need for a balance of work, play, and self-care. The human being is described as an open system. This means that all of our previous life experiences have an effect on how we behave now. One of Reilly's central beliefs was that play gives meaning to the daily life of a child. Play in childhood is seen as the primary vehicle for the cultivation of skills, abilities, interests, and habits of competition and cooperation needed for competence in adulthood (Parham & Primeau, 1997).

COTAs use play as the basis for many treatment sessions. A child's goals may be reached through the use of play, which can be used by the COTA to foster many developmental skills in children with any disability.

Biomechanical Frame of Reference

The biomechanical frame of reference frequently is used as the main approach with children who exhibit severe physical disabilities (Colangelo, 1993). It draws from theories in physics and physiology, and often is used in combination with other treatment approaches such as NDT. This frame of reference is used when the individual has neuromuscular or musculoskeletal dysfunction that interferes with her ability to maintain a posture. Thus, artificial supports are provided to substitute for the lack of postural control for functional activities. COTAs use this treatment approach when providing adaptive positioning equipment in the classroom and splints for a child.

Visual Perceptual Frame of Reference

There are many frames of reference that deal with visual perception but none dominates the field. Visual perception is the ability to interpret and use what is seen (Todd, 1993). Interpretation involves cognition that allows the child to put meaning to the stimulus. The continuous interaction of visual experience, intersensory feedback, and cognitive growth enhances the development of visual perceptual abilities (Hinojosa, Kramer, & Pratt, 1996). Many children with physical, developmental, or learning disabilities have difficulty using and interpreting visual information effectively in their environments. In the school setting, these children are described as having visual perceptual problems because they do not show adequate visual perceptual skills, yet they exhibit normal vision.

Coping Frame of Reference

The coping frame of reference recently was articulated by Zeitlin and Williamson in 1994 (Hinojosa, Kramer, & Pratt, 1996). Coping is the integration and application of developmental skills for functional living (Williamson, Szczepanski, & Zeitlin, 1993).

If a child can cope well, he will be able to learn effectively. This frame of reference focuses on the development and use of coping resources that enable a child to deal with present and future challenges and opportunities. Research has shown that children with disabilities have a more difficult time developing coping behaviors than their peers. This treatment approach can be used for children with a wide range of special needs. Because the outcome of any intervention is influenced by the child's coping competence, this approach should be incorporated into any intervention plan where it has been determined that a child has limited coping abilities (Williamson, Szczepanski, & Zeitlin, 1993). The coping frame of reference is meant for use in conjunction with other frames of reference.

Psychosocial Frame of Reference

The basis for the psychosocial frame of reference comes from a variety of theories that all address a child's emotional development. This theory considers innate temperament, attachment, peer interaction, play, coping ability, and environmental interaction. Children with behavioral or attention disorders have behaviors that interfere with their ability to function daily at home and school. The COTA may use this treatment approach when working with a child who has learning or language disabilities, autism or autistic-like features, or general developmental delays. The COTA's intervention with the child addresses and influences the child's total psychosocial function.

Chapter 2

School-Based Issues

IN 1975, THE U.S. CONGRESS PASSED A SERIES OF LAWS that sought to strengthen and improve the education of children with disabilities. The cumulative effect of this legislation resulted in the passage of the landmark statute, Education for All Handicapped Children Act (Public Law 94-142), which was amended and expanded in 1990 by the Individuals With Disabilities Education Act (IDEA, Public Law 101-476). The intent of IDEA is to assure that all children with disabilities receive a free, appropriate public education. Thus, special education is defined as specially designed instruction to meet the unique needs of a child with a disability. Special education is a series of individually designed services and supports.

An important part of this legislation made provisions for students with disabilities to receive educationally related services, which are support services needed to help a child with a disability benefit from special education. They can include physical therapy, adaptive physical education, speech therapy, and occupational therapy. All school-based therapy services are based on an educational model in which intervention seeks to enhance the student's ability to participate in the educational process. The educational model of service delivery is very different from the hospital-based medical model of service delivery. The medical model is a treatment approach that stresses decreasing the child's deficits. The educational model stresses using related services to support children in attaining their educational goals. School-based therapy is not meant to provide all the therapy a child will ever need in his or her lifetime to overcome a disability. Its purpose is to support the child in attaining maximum educational potential.

The Multifactored Evaluation

A school-age child is determined to be eligible for special education and related services through guidelines developed by the state and school district involved. Initially, a student will undergo a Multifactored Evaluation that includes descriptive data in all appropriate areas related to the suspected disability. This may include areas of health, vision, hearing, social and emotional states, adaptive behavior, cognition, academic performance, general intelligence, communication, and sensory-motor/motor abilities. Following the evaluation, the Individualized Education Plan (IEP) is written.

The Individualized Education Plan

The IEP, a written statement devised and implemented according to federal and state regulations, is the vehicle that directs and guides the development of meaningful educational experiences for each child with a disability. The IEP documents the school district's commitment to implement the educational program.

The IEP team members include the student's parents, teachers, and any related service providers who are or may need to be involved with the student. When appropriate, the student also is a member of his IEP team. Collaboration among all members of the team is essential for determining whether a specific motor service, physical therapy (PT), occupational therapy (OT), or adapted physical education (APE) is necessary to address the identified goals. If motor services are necessary for the student's educational experience, the team determines frequency, duration, and possible modes of service required. Although a student may exhibit deficits in an area associated with a specific service, the IEP team, not the individual service provider, decides what services are necessary. For example, if a student demonstrates deficits in fine-motor skills and hand function (the service area typically covered by OT), the IEP team, not the individual OTR, decides whether occupational therapy is necessary.

The IEP for each student must include a statement of: (1) the student's present level of development/function/educational performance; (2) annual goals, including short-term objectives that the student is expected to achieve in one school year; (3) methods for evaluation of each objective; (4) the specific special education and related services to be provided; (5) the projected date for initiation and duration of the services; and (6) the extent to which the child will be able to participate in regular educational programs.

Least Restrictive Environment

IDEA requires that children attend school in the least restrictive environment, which means that children with disabilities must be placed, to the maximum extent possible and appropriate, in regular educational settings with children who don't have disabilities.

Increasingly, students with disabilities, including those with severe disabilities, are being placed in general education classrooms in their own neighborhoods (Giangreco, Cloninger, & Iverson, 1993). This is called inclusion or mainstreaming, which often involves having related services such as occupational therapy provided in the general education setting, with the special education teacher consulting the classroom teacher about modifying materials and the curriculum.

Specialized classes are required only when the nature or severity of the disability precludes satisfactory achievement of the educational process in regular classes, even after supplemental aides and services have been utilized (Public Law 94-142, 1975). When indicated, a variety of specialized and preschool classrooms are provided for students with the following disabilities: learning, orthopedic, developmental, behavioral, and multiple. Every attempt should be made to mainstream students from specialized classrooms into classes or specific activities in which their developing peers typically participate. Examples of this might include but not be limited to mainstreaming for art, music, assemblies, class parties, lunch, and recess.

The Motor Team

For children whose motor limitations are adversely affecting their educational performance, positive results can be achieved when a team of motor specialists works in an integrated manner. The motor team may consist of OTs, COTAs, OTRs, PTAs, adapted physical educators, and physical educators. The motor team collaborates with all other educational team members to ensure that appropriate motor assessments and interventions are provided across all educational environments (Curatti, Kahl, & Eldridge, 1997).

The motor team model, as stated in the Ohio Motor Task Force Resource Guide (Curatti, Kahl, & Eldridge 1997), is a three-ring model that represents the three disciplines of physical therapy, occupational therapy, and adaptive physical education. Each segment of the three circles denotes areas examined by each individual discipline as well as areas of overlap between disciplines (Figure 1). This model is dynamic in nature and, therefore, ever changing depending upon the expertise and experience of the team. For example, positioning may be in the occupational-therapy-only segment if the physical therapy segment has no experience or expertise in positioning.

The Motor Team Model

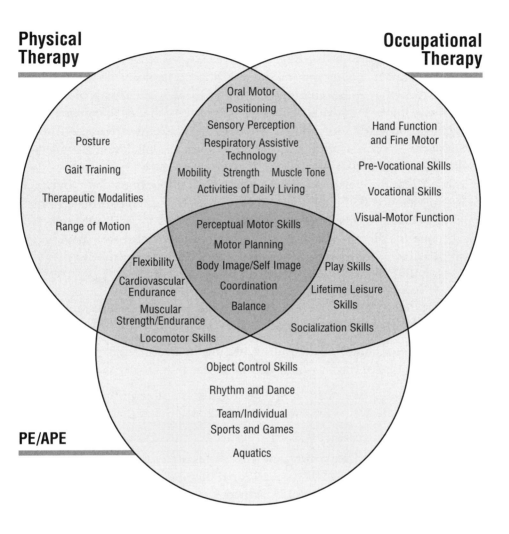

Physical Therapy

Occupational Therapy

PE/APE

Oral Motor
Positioning
Sensory Perception
Respiratory Assistive Technology
Mobility   Strength   Muscle Tone
Activities of Daily Living

Posture

Gait Training

Therapeutic Modalities

Range of Motion

Hand Function and Fine Motor

Pre-Vocational Skills

Vocational Skills

Visual-Motor Function

Perceptual Motor Skills
Motor Planning
Flexibility   Body Image/Self Image   Play Skills
Cardiovascular Endurance   Coordination   Lifetime Leisure Skills
Muscular Strength/Endurance   Balance
Locomotor Skills   Socialization Skills

Object Control Skills

Rhythm and Dance

Team/Individual Sports and Games

Aquatics

Figure 1.
The motor team model is dynamic and ever changing.
Ohio Motor Task Force Resource Guide, originated by Trish Curatti, M.S., P.T.; Dee Dee Kahl, M.S., OTR/L; Cynthia Eldridge, M.Ed., members.

Integrated Therapy

Integrated therapy is the type of intervention that takes place within the classroom, bathroom, lunchroom, or playground environment among the student's non-disabled peers (Johnson, 1996). This type of occupational therapy treatment enables the student to practice a new skill or use an adaptive technique in her environment with the other students present. The COTA may: (1) provide equipment or activities that enable the student to use maximum attention and participation in classroom activities; (2) need to adapt the environment in order for the student to function independently in the classroom; and (3) supervise a student's performance of a newly learned skill in the classroom amid all the added distractions that might cause interference. Although the goal of occupational therapy is to help the child function in the classroom, determining activities that are appropriate for meeting the therapy goals, as well as the environment that is most appropriate also is important (Johnson, 1996). These six methods of providing school-based therapy services are adapted from McWilliam (1995).

- *Individual pullout:* The student is removed from the classroom and returned after the therapy session.

- *Small group pullout:* The student and one or two peers is removed from the rest of the class and returned after the therapy session.

- *One-on-one in the classroom:* The student is treated in the corner of the classroom, possibly working on skills unrelated to the classroom routine.

- *Group activity:* The student and classmates are engaged in a group activity that addresses the occupational therapy needs of one or more students in the context of class activities.

- *Individual therapy during the classroom routine:* The student is supported during a classroom routine to develop specific skills related to classroom activities.

- *Consultation:* The therapy provider consults with the teacher to exchange information and expertise about a particular student's needs in the context of classroom activities.

The last three methods deliver therapy in an integrated manner with therapy treatments that support the education of the student. Integration of services helps promote greater team collaboration and improves outcomes for students because the skills are learned in the context of normal school routines. A combination of several types of intervention might be needed to meet a student's particular needs. The OTR and COTA need to look at each student's individual needs to determine the most appropriate type of intervention.

The Occupational Therapy Evaluation

The evaluation of a student's physical and developmental status is performed by a qualified OTR. However, in order to implement a pediatric plan of care effectively, the COTA must understand the purpose and process of evaluation that the OTR is likely to use in developing the plan of care. The COTA may contribute to the assessment process under the supervision of the OTR (AOTA, 1994b). For example, the COTA may perform supervised evaluations that are primarily focused on outcome data such as a standard score. When the COTA administers standardized tests, the OTR interprets the results of the data collected.

Pediatric occupational therapy evaluations typically require a medical and educational history, observations, and specific tests that are appropriate for the age of the child. An interview with the child's primary caregiver, teacher, or other adult working with the child is an excellent way to obtain a history. During a clinical observation of a child's neuro-motor status, the OTR observes many functional gross- and fine-motor skills while the child spontaneously plays or moves in the classroom environment. A functional evaluation of skills necessary in the schools includes observations of behavior/motivation, functional communication, manipulation skills needed for classroom activities, eating, self-care, and mobility. Following this, the child's muscle tone, range of motion, ocular-motor skills, reflexes, and balance reactions are tested through direct contact and physical handling.

A variety of evaluation tools are available to the pediatric OTR. The most commonly used evaluation tools include the *Pediatric Evaluation of Disability Inventory* (Haley, et al., 1992); the *Miller Assessment for Preschoolers* (Miller, 1988); the *DeGangi-Berk Test of Sensory Integration* (Berk & DeGangi, 1983); the *Erhardt Developmental Prehension Assessment* (Erhardt, 1989); the *Peabody Developmental Motor Scales* (Folio & Fewell, 1983); the *Bruininks-Oseretsky Test of Motor*

Performance (Bruininks, 1978); the *Beery-Buktenica Developmental Test of Visual-Motor Integration*, also known as the VMI (Beery, 1997); and the *School Function Assessment* (Coster, et al., 1998). Many tests are designed to give a score that compares the student's developmental age with others of the same age. This score may be used in determining eligibility for the school-based educational programs mentioned previously.

The format for a typical pediatric occupational therapy evaluation uses a subjective, objective, assessment, and plan (SOAP) guideline. Subjective findings include the history and observation sections. Objective findings include the details of any specialized tests as well as range of motion, strength, tone, fine-motor skills, and functional skills. Assessment includes the OTR's interpretation of the results, identification of abnormal findings, and functional deficits. Goals are developed, and a treatment plan is formed based on the assessment. The plan includes the recommended plan of care and suggestions for therapy. The entire IEP team, however, decides whether occupational therapy services are needed to support the student's education.

Role of the Certified Occupational Therapy Assistant

The COTA is an educated health-care provider who assists the OTR in the provision of occupational therapy. An OTR must supervise all phases and assume ultimate responsibility for the provision of these services. While the OTR may delegate all, some, or none of the treatment tasks to the COTA, the ultimate responsibility for the occupational therapy provided to the student—including evaluations—rests with the OTR (AOTA, 1997).

Supervision by the OTR fosters growth and development, assures appropriate utilization of training, encourages creativity and innovation, and provides guidance, support, encouragement, and respect while working toward a goal (AOTA, 1995).

Supervision of the COTA in the school system also varies according to the needs of the student, the COTA's level of education or experience, the comfort level of the supervising OTR, and the type of setting. However, the American Occupational Therapy Association (AOTA) states that COTAs at all levels of practice require at least general supervision by an OTR

(AOTA, 1997). General supervision requires at least monthly direct contact, with supervision available as needed by other methods (AOTA, 1995).

Supervision requirements also may be defined in state occupational therapy practice regulations, which take precedence over all other standards of practice. Therefore, all COTAs should be familiar with state laws and interpretations governing COTA practice and should take an active role in educating others about the role of the COTA. Two policies of the AOTA that establish standards for occupational therapy practitioners are the Code of Ethics (AOTA, 1994a) and the Standards of Practice for Occupational Therapy (AOTA, 1994b).

Competencies for COTAs in Educational Settings

Competence is a significant behavior performed in a specific setting to a specified standard (Davis, Anderson, & Jagger, 1979). An entry-level COTA or a COTA entering the school setting for the first time should demonstrate the following skills or competencies. The following competencies are adapted from Ratliffe and Tada (1997).

1. COTAs will appropriately handle and position a child with a severe motor disability to facilitate motor skills, socialization, functional skills, and participation in school activities. Examples of practical experiences to gain competency include:

   • Facilitate and inhibit movement in a child with severe disabilities during a therapy session.

   • Adapt positioning equipment to better meet the needs of the student.

   • Work with a specific student with severe disabilities in a group setting such as circle time.

2. COTAs will assist the OTR in taking measurements and observing the student's capabilities and needs. Examples of practical experiences to gain competency:

   • Take goniometric measurements of a student with contractures.

   • Observe limitation in range of motion.

3. COTAs will design and administer age-appropriate treatment activities based on the results of the OTR's assessment results and planned

intervention goals that foster integration of the student into the classroom, school, or community setting. Examples of practical experiences to gain competency:

- Plan a treatment session based on occupational therapy goals.
- Organize the treatment area or equipment to prepare for a treatment session.
- Adapt activities based on the student's changing needs or circumstances.

4. COTAs will have adequate written communication skills for gathering relevant information and providing documentation of service. Examples of practical experiences to gain competency:

- Write a progress note or SOAP note that documents the student's current level of performance or treatment session.
- Complete required paperwork for billing or documenting provided services to third-party payers or administrators.
- Communicate to the supervising therapist regarding the student's needs.

5. COTAs will be creative in using available resources including space, equipment, toys, peers, and learning materials to assist in therapy activities. Examples of practical experiences to gain competency:

- Adapt existing positioning equipment for improved access or position for the student.
- Create a new piece of equipment to help the student with positioning or mobility skills.
- Plan for or rearrange furniture or equipment to promote improved access to classroom, recess, or therapy services.

6. COTAs will demonstrate understanding of family support principles by encouraging family advocacy, facilitating family involvement in the team process, and respecting family rights and perspectives. Examples of practical experiences to gain competency:

- Interact with individuals from different agencies involved with the student.
- Research community support to help the family solve a particular problem.

7. COTAs will understand the various types of team relationships and interact collaboratively with team members to implement therapy activities, participate in planning meetings, and assist in developing goals and strategies for integrated inclusive education. Examples of practical experiences to gain competency:

   • Participate actively in a team meeting.

   • Assist the OTR in writing IEP goals and objectives.

8. COTAs will have adequate oral communication skills with which to foster relationships, and will work collaboratively with other team members. Examples of practical experiences to gain competency:

   • During the day, observe and interact with other team members (e.g., PT, speech-language pathologist, teacher, and APE teacher).

   • Plan collaborative activities with other team members.

9. COTAs will understand cultural influences on attitudes, family adaptation, and program development for children with disabilities. Examples of practical experiences to gain competency:

   • Research a cultural perspective different from the COTA's own.

   • Present an in-service workshop to the staff regarding cultural issues.

10. COTAs will understand how special education teachers interact with students in various educational environments such as self-contained classrooms, mainstreamed situations, and inclusive classrooms. Examples of practical experiences to gain competency:

   • Work with students in different types of classrooms or settings.

   • Visit and observe different educational settings.

11. COTAs will explain how they might interact with special educators in the various environments described above to provide integrated services to students. Examples of practical experiences to gain competency:

   • Plan intervention that is directly related to the educational goals of a student.

   • Collaborate with a special education teacher to plan an integrated group or individual therapy session.

- Consult with a special education teacher about one or more students with motor needs.

12. COTAs will know and act according to professional ethical standards in accordance with local laws governing the provision of occupational therapy services to students in educational settings. Examples of practical experiences to gain competency:

   - Give a presentation to the staff regarding the supervision of COTAs by OTRs.

   - Discuss with an OTR supervisor ethical issues that arise when providing treatment to students.

   - Assist with data collection and evaluation under the supervision of an OTR (AOTA, 1994b).

Chapter 3

Quick Reference to Pediatric Disorders

Arthrogryposis Multiplex Congenita (AMC)

Arthrogryposis multiplex congenita (AMC) is a nonprogressive, congenital disorder present at birth that is characterized by fibrous ankylosis of multiple joints, multiple joint contractures, and muscle weakness. The generalized fixation of joints may be due to a variety of changes in the spinal cord, muscles, or connective tissue. The incidence of mental retardation is no greater for this population than for the general population. Arthrogryposis occurs in approximately 1 out of every 3,000 births.

Five classic signs of AMC include (a) featureless involved extremities that are cylindrical with absent skin creases; (b) rigidity of joints; (c) dislocation of joints, especially the hips; (d) atrophy and absence of muscles or muscle groups; and (e) intact sensation, although deep-tendon reflexes may be diminished or absent.

Associated Problems

Because of the contractures, hip dislocation or subluxation can occur. Some extremities such as the elbows and knee joints may have few or no features, and some muscle groups may be absent. Associated abnormalities include scoliosis, a cleft palate, facial abnormalities, and failure to thrive.

Treatment

Treatment includes: (1) exercises to increase range of motion, improve mobility, and increase muscle strength; (2) positioning and splinting to decrease deformity; and (3) adaptive equipment to promote functional skills.

Autism

Like mental retardation, autism is a brain-based developmental disability with multiple causes. Autism differs from mental retardation in that its characteristic feature is not a delay in development, but a series of striking deviations from normal development. Autism involves disturbances in cognition, interpersonal communication, social interactions, and behavior. Often, the student with autism demonstrates obsessive, ritualistic, stereotypical, and rigid behaviors.

Impaired social skills can appear as a lack of interest in the feelings of others and the absence of eye contact. Communication disorders may be present as delays and deviations in both expressive and receptive communication. About half of the students with autism remain mute. Those who develop language do not use it creatively or spontaneously. They tend to repeat phrases and long commercial jingles. Obsessive rituals and strict adherence to routines are common in students with autism. For example, there may be rigid insistence on eating the same foods at the same time every day and on sitting in the same spot at the table. Young children with autism may show intense attachment to unusual objects such as a piece of plastic rather than a cuddly item such as a teddy bear. Frequently, students with autism become upset and have intense temper tantrums if anything interferes with these rituals and preoccupations. Stereotyped movements and self-stimulating behaviors such as rocking, hand waving, arm flapping, head banging, and other forms of self-injurious behavior are common in students with autism who have low IQs (Pauls & Reed, 1996).

Associated Problems

About 70% of students with autism have mental retardation: 35% of those students have mild retardation, 15% have moderate retardation, and 20% have severe or profound retardation. Twenty-five percent fall in borderline-to-normal range of intelligence, and about 5% have high IQs (Minshew & Payton, 1988).

Other associated problems include a range of sensory disturbances such as oversensitivity to certain sounds, indifference to pain, and a preference for certain sensations. Most students with autism are clumsy and have some abnormalities of posture and movement.

Treatment

Treatment of a student with autism includes the fostering of normal development, promotion of learning, reduction of rigidity, elimination of maladaptive behaviors, and alleviation of family distress. These goals are best met through a comprehensive educational program with behavior management that includes a highly structured educational setting, language training, behavioral interventions, positive social experiences, and intensive parental involvement.

Brachial Plexus Injury (BPI)

A *brachial plexus injury* is one that involves damage to nerves that control muscles in the shoulder, arm, and hand. Any or all of these muscles could become paralyzed. Most brachial plexus injuries occur during birth when the baby's neck and shoulders are stretched too far apart, thus damaging or tearing the nerves of the brachial plexus. Many babies with brachial plexus injury are larger than average at birth; however, newborns of any size can sustain a brachial plexus injury if these nerves are damaged.

There are four types of nerve injuries—avulsion, rupture, neuroma, and praxis. An avulsion occurs when a nerve is torn from the spine. A nerve that is torn elsewhere is a rupture. A neuroma is a nerve that has tried to heal itself, but scar tissue has grown around the injury and is putting pressure on the injured nerve. In a praxis injury, a nerve has been damaged but not torn. Praxis injuries heal by themselves, and within several months, the paralysis disappears.

Erb's Palsy is the term used when the injury involves an upper root palsy (C5-C6) of the brachial plexus. Erb's Klumpke Palsy is the term used when the entire brachial plexus (C5-T1) is affected. Klumpke Palsy is an injury to C8-T1 and is less common.

Associated Problems

Children with BPI are affected differently depending on the type of injury, but all have some limitations in the use of the affected arm. A child with BPI usually will present an internally rotated and adducted arm with some wrist flexion. Some children may experience no muscle control or sensation (feeling) in the affected arm or hand. Others can move their arms but have little control over their wrists and hands, while yet other children can use their hands well but cannot use their shoulders or elbow muscles effectively. School functioning becomes a secondary challenge to this disability.

Treatment

Treatment of a child with BPI starts at infancy. Daily exercises help keep the muscles and joints moving normally while splints are used for proper positioning. Surgery may help children who have lost significant arm function. Treatment in the school setting involves adapting the child's classroom environment, providing adaptive equipment, splinting, and educating the teaching staff. Most children with BPI are in regular educational settings with no other limitations than that of the physical involvement of the arm.

Cerebral Palsy (CP)

Cerebral palsy is a group of nonprogressive upper motor neuron disorders manifested by motor dysfunction. CP is a broad term used to describe a number of motor disorders occurring before age five. CP can occur because of prenatal developmental abnormalities (during pregnancy), perinatal abnormalities (during birth), or postnatal abnormalities (after birth). There are several types of CP. *Spastic CP* is the most common type and represents about 70% of the cases. The spasticity is due to upper motor neuron involvement and may affect motor function mildly or severely. *Hemiplegia* denotes involvement of both upper and lower extremities on one side; the arm usually is more involved than the leg. *Paraplegia* denotes involvement of both lower extremities. *Quadriplegia* denotes involvement of all extremities to a similar degree. *Diplegia* refers to a quadriplegia with mild involvement of the upper extremities.

Athetoid or dyskinetic CP occurs in about 20% of the cases and results from basal ganglia involvement. It is characterized by purposeless, uncontrollable movements and muscle tension. The movements increase with emotional tension and disappear during sleep.

Ataxic CP is uncommon (10% of the cases) and results from involvement of the cerebellum or its pathways. It is characterized by poor balance, incoordination, and a wide-based gait.

Mixed types of CP occur in about 10% of the cases. The most common form is spasticity with athetosis. The less common mixed type is ataxia and athetosis.

Associated Problems

Students with CP may have a number of oculo-motor problems including strabismus, homonymous hemianopsia, and nystagmus. Strabismus indicates a *lazy eye*, homonymous hemianopsia indicates a visual field cut, and nystagmus indicates poor coordination of the eye muscles. Because of the abnormal tone and poor control of the muscles of the face, mouth, and respiratory system, students with CP may have difficulty with feeding and communication. Mental retardation occurs in 40% to 60% of the cases and is most common in children with quadriplegia, rigidity, and atonia (Pauls & Reed, 1996). Seizures occur in about 50% of the students. Communication difficulties are due to poor oral-motor control, central language dysfunction, hearing impairment, or cognitive deficits.

Treatment

Treatment in the school setting includes assisting the child in participating in the educational process. This may include maximizing development of normal movement patterns, facilitating oral-motor function, preventing contractures, increasing postural tone in trunk musculature, promoting full range of motion in extremities, increasing muscle control, developing smoothly coordinated and automatic reactions, providing adaptive equipment, and maximizing function in the school setting.

Deaf-Blindness

A student with *deaf-blindness* has both an auditory impairment and a visual impairment that are present from birth or acquired in infancy. The degree of loss is quite variable. There are two types of hearing loss, conductive and sensorineural. Conductive hearing loss is due to middle-ear dysfunction and is structural in origin. Sensorineural hearing loss is due to neurological factors that involve the inner ear and/or auditory nerve.

In childhood, the causes of blindness are many and varied. The most common congenital causes are intrauterine infections and malformations. Intrauterine infections such as rubella and toxoplasmosis could cause severe retinal damage. Malformations of the visual system range from optic nerve hypoplasia to cerebral malformations.

Associated Problems

In addition to developmental delays, the child with deaf-blindness may exhibit unusual behaviors. Self-stimulatory behaviors may include pressing the eye, blinking forcefully, rolling the head, and swaying the body. Self-stimulatory behaviors occur most commonly when the child is bored or tired.

Treatment

Treatment includes using familiar daily routines; hands-on learning; movements that increase awareness and skill; and facilitation of motor, communication, and visual skills.

Down Syndrome

Down Syndrome is a chromosomal disorder in which extra genetic material results in hypotonia, musculoskeletal differences, and mental retardation. The most common type, found in 95% of the cases, is called *nondisjunction trisomy 21* because there is a third 21st chromosome present in all cells. Other types are translocation, where the 21st chromosome breaks off during cell division and attaches to another chromosome, and mosaicism, where the faulty cell division occurs after fertilization with only some of the cells having the extra chromosome.

The characteristic appearance of a child with Down Syndrome may include hypotonia, joint hyperflexibility, a flat facial profile, external ear anomalies, short stature, excessive skin around the neck, and a simian crease (single midpalmar crease).

The incidence of Down Syndrome is about 1 in 700 live births (Batshaw & Perret, 1992). There is an association between Down Syndrome and advanced maternal age. The risk of a 35- to 39-year-old woman having a child with Down Syndrome is approximately 6.5 times that of a 20- to 24-year-old. This figure climbs to 20.5 times for mothers between 40 and 44 years of age because nondisjunction of the cells is far more likely to occur in older parents (Batshaw & Perret, 1992).

Associated Problems

In addition to the distinctive physical features, students with Down Syndrome have some level of mental retardation. The degree of mental retardation varies tremendously. Virtually all children with Down Syndrome have some vision problem, including refractive errors (70%), strabismus (50%), nystagmus (35%), and cataracts (3%). Hearing problems resulting from narrow ear canals coupled with a subtle immune deficiency predispose these children to recurrent middle-ear infections. Of children with Down Syndrome, 60% to 90% have a mild-to-moderate conductive hearing loss resulting from chronic middle-ear infections. Gastrointestinal abnormalities occur in 15% of students with Down Syndrome (Batshaw & Perret, 1992). These include small bowel obstruction, esophageal malformations, and imperforate anus. Forty percent of students with Down Syndrome have congenital heart defects. Many of the heart defects can lead to heart failure and usually require open-heart surgery in infancy.

In later childhood, additional medical problems may develop, the most common being obesity, short stature, hypothyroidism, seizures, and joint dislocations. The most common of these are short stature and obesity. More than half of children with Down Syndrome demonstrate excessive weight gain from overeating and inactivity (Pueschel, et al., 1987).

Partial dislocation of the upper spine (atlantooccipital or atlantoaxial subluxation) occurs in about 15% of students with Down Syndrome (Pueschel & Scola, 1987). Because these dislocations can lead to spinal cord compression, they must be detected early. Symptoms of spinal cord compression include a head tilt, increasing clumsiness, limping or refusing to walk, and weakness of an arm. Due to this concern, an X ray of the neck is advisable before the student participates in contact sports or gymnastics. Surgical fusion of the upper vertebral column may be needed, if the student is found to have this.

Treatment

Treatment focuses on improving muscle strength, especially the antigravity muscles, and facilitating attainment of developmental skills and effective oral-motor function.

Juvenile Rheumatoid Arthritis (JRA)

Juvenile rheumatoid arthritis (JRA) is arthritis that begins before age sixteen. Arthritis is defined as swelling and limitation of motion of a joint with some combination of heat, pain, and tenderness. JRA tends to affect both large and small joints, which may result in interference with growth and development. Common features of JRA include joint inflammation, joint contractures, joint damage, and altered growth. The cause is unknown. Some possible factors include infection, autoimmunity, trauma, and genetic predisposition.

Associated Problems

JRA is divided into three subtypes, each with its own associated problems. The systemic type is characterized by daily fever and other systemic inflammations. There is pain and inflammation in many joints, with gait dysfunction and decreased performance of activities of daily living if upper extremities are involved. There usually is multisystem or organ involvement such as pericarditis, myocarditis, or hepatosplenomegaly.

The pauciarticular type presents pain and inflammation in four joints or less. This type affects females 4:1, and 70% of the students will have no functional impairment after fifteen years.

The polyarticular type involves five or more joints with females being affected 3:1. Symmetrical joint involvement is seen with knees, wrist, and ankles representing the most common pattern of involvement.

Treatment

Treatment focuses on attaining and maintaining joint mobility, range of motion, and muscle strength—which assist in controlling pain—as well as splinting, providing adaptive equipment, and promoting proper joint alignment.

Mental Retardation (MR)

Mental retardation (MR) is defined as subaverage intellectual ability that is present from birth or early infancy and manifested by abnormal development and associated with difficulties in learning and social adaptation.

Mental retardation is classified as mild (IQ 55–69), moderate (40–54), severe (25–39), and profound (0–24).

In 80% of the cases, the cause of MR is unknown, but more than 200 conditions are known to cause retardation. Factors causing MR may occur in the prenatal, perinatal, and postnatal periods.

Associated Problems

Students with MR may show motor-control problems including muscle weakness, joint limitation, delayed developmental milestones, and abnormal tone. They also may have sensory and perceptual problems, seizures, oral-motor difficulties, receptive and expressive language problems, and behavior difficulties.

Treatment

Treatment should focus on the development and reinforcement of appropriate adaptive behaviors that are interesting, fun, and pleasurable. Therapy targets specific areas of deficits and focuses on improving functional outcomes. Therapy can include developing sensory integration skills, oral-motor control and skills, and postural balance and control. Therapy also can focus on using behavior modification techniques to reinforce motivation and reduce self-injurious and self-stimulation behaviors.

Muscular Dystrophy (MD)

Muscular dystrophy (MD) is a general term for a number of hereditary, progressive, and degenerative disorders affecting skeletal or voluntary muscles that control movement. The different types are distinguished primarily on clinical grounds. The types of MD include Becker muscular dystrophy, limb-girdle muscular dystrophy, facioscapulohumeral, mitochondrial myopathies, and Duchenne muscular dystrophy (DMD).

Duchenne muscular dystrophy (DMD) is the most common childhood muscular dystrophy and hereditary neuromuscular disease with onset usually before age six. Because it is an X-linked recessive disorder, only boys are affected. Proximal muscle weakness causes waddling gait, toe-walking, lordosis, frequent falls, and difficulty in standing up and climbing stairs. Pseudohypertrophy (enlargement) of the calf muscles occurs due to fatty and fibrous infiltration of the muscles. Progression is steady, and most students are in wheelchairs by ages ten to twelve.

Associated Problems

Cardiac involvement is common in DMD. The average IQ of a student with DMD is one standard deviation below the mean, indicating mild mental retardation. Flexion contractures and scoliosis ultimately occur due to weakness and increased time spent in the wheelchair. Most students with DMD die by age twenty, usually because of respiratory failure alone or secondary to infection.

Treatment

Treatment is based on the problems of the individual child but may include range of motion and positioning to prevent deformity and contractures, maintaining ambulation, teaching of energy conservation techniques, and maintaining functional abilities. Prolonged ambulation is possible through surgical techniques, orthopedic devices, and physical therapy. Exercise programs should be limited to active assisted range of motion (AAROM) and passive range of motion (PROM) because strengthening exercises could fatigue the muscles excessively.

Rett Syndrome

Although *Rett syndrome* is a neurological disorder found exclusively in females, it is an inherited disorder that's presumed to be X-linked and lethal to males. There are four stages of this degenerative syndrome. Muscle-tone abnormalities occur and gross-motor skills decrease as spasticity and apraxia increase. Reaction time is slow, and students with Rett syndrome may have difficulty initiating movement.

Associated Problems

As the student regresses, stereotypical hand movements (clapping, wringing, clenching) that are involuntary increase with intent. There is a loss of functional mobility due to spasticity, ataxia, apraxia, and compensatory spinal rigidity. Spatial disorientation in the upright position may cause leaning backward, forward, or laterally. Oral-motor skills are affected, with a regression in feeding skills and drooling occurring. Behavior changes occur with the student demonstrating autistic-like behavior, dementia, and retardation.

Treatment

Treatment should focus on developing, maintaining, or regaining ambulation and transitional skills. Treatment to elicit righting and equilibrium responses as well as techniques to prevent or reduce deformities also are indicated.

Spina Bifida

Spina bifida is the most common neural tube defect in which there is a defective closure of the vertebral column. There are two classifications of spina bifida, occulta and cystica. Spina bifida *occulta* is the mildest form and is present in 40% of the American population. Most individuals with this condition have no problems, and it often presents as a tuft of hair in the lower lumbar spine.

Spina bifida *cystica* is a defect in which the meninges have pushed through the openings in the unclosed vertebrae, forming an external sac, or cyst, on the child's back called a *meningocele*. There are two types of spina bifida cystica: meningocele and myelomeningocele. *Meningocele* is the mildest and the rarest. The sac does not involve the nerve roots or spinal cord, which are normally left intact. *Myelomeningocele* is the most severe and occurs in 96% of the students with spina bifida cystica. In this type, the sac does contain nerve roots and often the spinal cord itself, thus causing paraplegia at the level of the defect.

Spina bifida appears to be a genetic disorder that is affected by environmental factors. The exact relationship is unknown.

Associated Problems

Seventy to 90% of students with spina bifida have hydrocephalus, the abnormal accumulation of cerebral spinal fluid (CSF) in the cranial vault. Another related condition is the Arnold-Chiari malformation (Chiari II). This is considered to be the cause of hydrocephalus in most students with spina bifida. This malformation is caused when the posterior cerebellum herniates inferiorly through the foramen magnum causing a displacement of the brainstem structures in a caudal direction. The CSF from the fourth ventricle may become obstructed by these abnormally situated structures, and the flow of CSF through the foramen magnum may be disrupted. This results in the enlargement of the ventricles or hydrocephalus.

In general, infants with hydrocephalus require a shunting procedure several days after the spinal opening is surgically closed. In this procedure, CSF from the enlarged ventricular system is diverted to another place in the body where it can be better absorbed. Most frequently a ventriculo-peritoneal (V-P) shunt is used, through which the fluid is drained into the infant's abdominal cavity. The procedure involves placing a small, plastic catheter into one of the enlarged ventricles. This catheter runs under the skin of the neck and chest and into the abdominal cavity. Extra tubing is left in the abdomen so that as the child grows, the catheter can uncoil without getting clogged.

Once placed, the shunt may become blocked. Symptoms of a blocked shunt include headaches, vomiting, and irritability. A second potential complication of a V-P shunt is infection. In this case, the student may become febrile and lethargic and begin vomiting.

Motor paralysis results from the spinal cord malformation. The motor level is defined as the lowest intact functional neuromuscular segment. The higher the spinal cord malformation in the spine the more limited the student will be.

Other associated problems are musculoskeletal deformities. The cause of the deformities includes muscle imbalance, progressive neurologic dysfunction, habitually assumed postures after birth, reduced joint motion, and deformities after fractures. Spinal curvatures and humps occur in almost 90% of students with spina bifida. These deformities include scoliosis, a spinal curve; kyphosis, a spinal hump; and kyphoscoliosis, a combination of both conditions. Other consequences of muscle imbalance are a club foot and hip dislocation.

Bladder and bowel dysfunction are present in virtually all students with myelomeningocele, regardless of their level of spinal cord lesion or paralysis. This is because messages from nerves for bladder and bowel function are conveyed through the second sacral-fourth sacral (S2-S4) level of the spinal cord. Even those students with sacral lesions and normal leg movement often have bladder and bowel problems.

Skin sores or decubital ulcers often occur in students with myelomeningocele. For most of these students, the weight-bearing surfaces of their bodies (e.g., feet, buttocks) are not sensitive to pain. Thus, sores become a problem when students are immobile and sustain injuries that they do not feel. Management of this problem should be anticipatory: Replace tight-fitting shoes or braces, avoid hot baths or crawling on rough or hot surfaces, perform pressure reliefs during class, and modify the wheelchair with an appropriate cushion.

Approximately 15% of students with myelomeningocele have seizures, and the most common cause of the seizures is usually associated with a blocked shunt.

Cognitive dysfunction is more prevalent in students with hydrocephalus. Without hydrocephalus or with uncomplicated hydrocephalus, the student will fall within the normal range of intelligence.

Treatment

Treatment focuses on improving functional posture for sitting or standing, preventing skin breakdown, fitting with orthotics and range-of-motion exercises, preventing contractures and fractures by administering a standing program, and providing equipment for maximum mobility.

Traumatic Brain Injury/Head Injury

Most head trauma in children is minor and not associated with persisting deficits (Batshaw & Perret, 1992). However, *craniocerebral trauma* and its complications are a leading cause of injury and death in children. Injury to the central nervous system often results in residual impairment of physical, cognitive, and emotional functions. A skull fracture may cause a subdural hematoma (a collection of blood beneath the dura mater) or an epidural hematoma (a collection of blood between the dura mater and the skull). Even when obvious physical problems are minimal, neuropsychological deficits may lead to chronic academic, behavioral, and interpersonal difficulties.

Head injury is the second most common form of trauma in children—especially with boys between the ages of one and fifteen—that requires hospitalization. Frequently occurring causes of head injury are car and bicycle accidents, falls, diving accidents, birth injuries, contact sports, and child abuse.

Brain injury is defined as trauma sufficient to result in a change in level of consciousness and/or an anatomical abnormality of the brain. When a coma results because of a brain injury, the duration and severity of the coma indicates the seriousness of the brain injury. There are several scales that are used to rate the severity of the injury, and the most frequently used scale is the Glasgow Coma Score (GCS).

Associated Problems

Students with brain injuries often experience motor deficits. The site of the brain injury determines the type of motor dysfunction. Spasticity, ataxia, and tremor are common motor abnormalities.

Feeding disorders often accompany motor deficits. Food intake may decrease if the ability to obtain food or to eat is compromised because of impaired motor skills or swallowing problems.

Vision and hearing can be affected by traumatic brain injury. The most common vision problem is diplopia (double vision), which is caused by eye-muscle palsy. Hearing loss is a less common problem following head injury. If present, it usually is unilateral and caused by direct physical trauma to the temporal bone.

If the left hemisphere of the brain is damaged, speech and language deficits are likely. Usually when language is disordered, cognition also is affected. Cognitive deficits may include problems with attention, concentration, memory, impaired judgment, and distractibility.

Treatment

Treatment includes activities to prevent contractures, as well as range of motion, active exercise, motor learning, oral-motor exercises, and behavior-management techniques.

Chapter 4

Therapy Ideas
and Suggestions

ESTABLISHING RAPPORT AND TRUST with the student is important. Initially, approach the student slowly, starting at eye level so as not to intimidate the young student. Allow the student to become comfortable with your presence. Although each therapy session will have predetermined goals, the key is to make therapy seem like play. The challenge is to work on therapy goals as the unknowing student plays a game or engages in a fun activity. Toys and play motivate children and make therapy enjoyable for you and the student. Understanding play in the context of child development and cultivating our own playfulness and adaptability can help make therapy more fun as well as more effective and productive for us and the children. (Ratliffe, 1998).

During therapy, remember to pay attention to how much area your hands are covering on the student. Pay attention to the amount of force or weight shift that is required to have an effect on the student. A small excursion of movement by the COTA can result in a large weight shift for the student. For example, the position of a student seated on the COTA's lap could be changed if the COTA merely lifts one of her legs.

Treatment of Students with Hypotonicity

The most common diagnoses of students with hypotonicity are Down Syndrome, muscular dystrophy, spinal muscle atrophy, and general developmental delay. Students with cerebral palsy can present with hypotonicity, but often it is a precursor either to hypertonicity or athetosis. Because most students with hypotonicity have problems with control at midranges of movement, many of the treatment suggestions focus on increasing midrange control. These suggestions include working on transfers and transitional movements such as prone to quadruped, sit to stand, stand to tall kneel, and tall kneel to sit.

Another area of weakness seen in students with hypotonicity is decreased postural stability or proximal stability. By improving proximal stability, distal mobility can be improved (stability before mobility). In other words, the student needs to have strength and stability in the shoulder before he can effectively use his hand for prewriting or writing activities. Proximal stability is needed through the shoulders and hips (more proximal joints) and the trunk. Weight bearing through the trunk or extremities in a variety of positions also stimulates postural stability. Facilitated weight shifting will assist a student in developing co-contraction around proximal joints so that independent weight shift can be accomplished (Ratliffe, 1998). An example of an activity to improve a student's proximal stability would be placing the student in the wheelbarrow position (hold the lower extremities and the child weight bears through the upper extremities) and having her walk across the room. Or, by having the student push the assistant on a swing or a scooter, the student is weight bearing through his upper extremities and improving his postural stability. Another easy way to have the student work on stability activities is to routinely have her push or pull open doors that are encountered in the school, to and from the restroom, office, or cafeteria.

A student with hypotonicity may need tactile input to enable him to produce more energetic movement. Techniques, such as tapping, brushing, vibrating, rubbing, or providing deep pressure to a muscle or the skin have been found to increase motor response (Ratliffe, 1998).

Because students with hypotonicity require more time to process and respond, deep input or pressure, often in the form of joint approximation, often is given by the assistant. After giving the deep input, the COTA should back off and use light touch and guidance to facilitate movement in order to allow the student to be an active participant in the treatment session. This is because students with hypotonicity tend to sink into their support surfaces (e.g., desks, tables, the COTA's hands).

Treatment of Students with Hypertonicity

The most common diagnosis of students with hypertonicity is cerebral palsy (CP). Many students with CP are dominated by strong extensor tone. This presents as neck hyperextension that causes poor head control and poor visual skills; trunk extension resulting in the inability to weight shift; and lower extremity extension with scissoring of the legs due to increased tone of the hamstrings, adductors, and gastrocnemius.

Stereotypical movements seen in students with hypertonicity include: flips to roll; rolls to toys instead of crawls; W-sits; bunny hops instead of creeping; and walks on toes with decreased weight shift and trunk rotation.

Treatment of students with hypertonicity focuses on relaxing and optimizing the effects of lowering the tone in order to use muscles more effectively. This is achieved by a combination of proper positioning and hands-on techniques that may include sensory integration (SI) and neurodevelopmental treatment (NDT), as well as gentle rocking and rhythmic movements.

The NDT approach uses handling by the therapist or assistant at the student's head, shoulders, pelvis, or hips. These proximal points are called *key points of control* where abnormal movements can be inhibited and normal postural reactions facilitated.

Range-of-motion exercises often are indicated to prevent contractures and enable the students to tolerate a variety of positioning equipment. By providing a variety of movement patterns, the COTA can minimize the risk of the student developing contractures and joint deformity. Generalized activities to improve gross-motor developmental skills also may be incorporated in the treatment plan, as well as mobility skills and activities to promote balance reactions.

The student with hypertonicity usually demonstrates poor balance and equilibrium because of poor postural reflexes. Often, a student with severe spasticity will have only a few positions that can be regularly assumed independently. Treatment should focus on providing varied movement patterns and promoting initiation of movement. Movements of the student with hypertonicity are frequently ruled by persistent reflex patterns that have not been integrated into mature patterns of movement. It is important for the COTA to be aware of these reflex patterns and focus treatment on inhibiting abnormal reflex patterns. Avoiding positions that stimulate abnormal reflex activity is essential to helping students attain and maintain functional positions. Encouraging midline orientation of the head by helping the child look forward rather than to the side can help avoid asymmetry.

Treatment of Students with Fluctuating Tone (Athetosis)

Some students with the diagnosis of cerebral palsy (CP) present with fluctuating tone. Athetosis occurs when muscles on both sides of the joints cannot be coordinated to stabilize the joint. Because the students cannot stabilize their movements, especially in the midranges of the joint's movement, they tend to move from one extreme of the range to the other. When students demonstrate spasticity and athetosis, they are especially at risk for developing contractures. This is because they tend to *fix* their posture at one extreme of their range and have a difficult time moving out of that position. Persistence of early reflexes usually is seen in the student with athetosis.

Treatment of the student with athetosis focuses on maintaining symmetrical posturing. This is very important so that the student can optimize functional and social skills, and the visual system will develop optimally. Symmetry, or midline control, can be achieved with positioning and adaptive equipment as well as with the hands-on therapy techniques mentioned previously. Treatment should first begin proximally and then, as control is attained, the distal structures can be addressed. Slow and steady movements of the assistant can help the student regulate movements in a more controlled manner. Compression to foster joint approximation and vibratory stimuli are indicated when treating the student with athetosis.

Carrying the Student

Small students with disabilities can be carried and lifted by one person. However, larger students will require a two-person lift, transfer, or carry. Proper body mechanics must be stressed whenever instructing others in the previously mentioned techniques.

A student with hypertonia should be carried in positions that inhibit the abnormal reflex postures. This can be achieved in many ways. One way is by carrying the student face-forward, keeping the hips and knees flexed as well as the neck slightly flexed, if the student is dominated by strong extensor tone (Figure 2). This position allows the student to interact with the environment and work on midline orientation. When strong adductor tone dominates, the student can be carried on the side of the caregiver, straddling the caregiver's hip. Placing each leg astride inhibits the adductor tone. Another carry involves the caregiver placing his arm between the legs of the student while supporting the trunk with another arm (Figure 2).

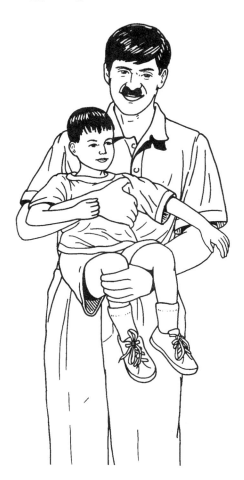

Figure 2. One of the preferred ways to carry a small student with hypertonicity.

A student with hypotonia should be carried in a way that fully supports the head, trunk, and extremities. Being supported and resting over a caregiver's shoulder allows the child to lift her head up briefly and observe the surroundings.

Careful attention should be paid to the extremities when moving or carrying any student. Those with osteoporosis could experience fractures if an unsupported extremity hits the edge of a chair, table, or piece of adaptive equipment.

Feeding

Children with significant motor impairments often exhibit oral-motor/feeding delays. Examples of children who have motor dysfunction that can affect feeding are those with CP, autism, prematurity, or genetic syndromes. An optimal feeding program at school allows the students to experience optimal oral-feeding experiences along with their positive social and developmental ramifications, as well as receive the necessary combination of nutrients and fluids to help them grow and remain healthy (Eicher, 1998).

Oral-motor skill acquisition follows a developmental progression similar to that of other motor skills (Eicher, 1998). For example, a child whose skills are at a seven-month level of development will not have the neurological maturity to chew finger food or other hard solids adequately. Oral skills follow a hierarchical sequence, and the student must progress through every stage of feeding without skipping any stages. Because of this, children do not progress from bottle to finger foods without experiencing purees (see Stages of Oral-Motor Development, page 6).

The act of feeding requires a high level of oral-motor control and coordination superimposed on adequate trunk alignment and support (Eicher, 1998). Feeding is best accomplished with the head and trunk in proper alignment and the hips, knees, and ankles at a 90-degree angle with the feet positioned flat on a stable base. Predominance of extensor tone throughout the body will decrease the student's oral-pharyngeal control.

Many specific feeding problems exist in students with motor impairments. Persistent suckling is very common in students who have an exaggerated suckle reflex due to the delayed inhibition of primitive reflex patterns.

This exaggerated reflex interferes with successful spoon-feeding because the food rides off the tongue. Lack of chewing occurs when oral-motor skills are immature and the student is unable to process chunks or lumps of food. Rather than chewing, the student may push the lumps into the cheek to prevent choking or gagging which, along with coughing, are natural protective responses aimed at keeping the oral airway clear (Eicher, 1998).

Treatment of Feeding Problems

When managing feeding problems at school, the COTA must first ensure proper positioning during feeding. To provide a stable base, the student should be firmly supported through the hips and trunk during feeding. Many children need to be positioned in a wheelchair or adapted chair to provide the optimal position for feeding tasks. The COTA will need to ensure that the student maintains an appropriate position during lunch and educate the student's teacher on the importance of this. Next, the head and neck should be aligned in a neutral position, which decreases extension through the oral musculature while maintaining an open airway (Eicher, 1998). A chin-tuck position generally is best for feeding.

The COTA can facilitate optimal oral-motor function during mealtime. For example, spoon placement with gentle pressure on the mid-tongue region can help remind the student to keep the tongue inside the mouth. Placing food laterally between the upper and lower molars can enhance chewing. Food textures can be manipulated to facilitate safe, controlled swallowing (Gisel, 1994). Thickening of liquids allows more time for the student to control the bolus and initiate a swallow by slowing the flow rate. Thickening agents such as Thickit, potato flakes, and instant pudding powders can change any thin liquid into a more optimal consistency. In addition, almost any food can be finely chopped or pureed to a texture that the student can competently manage.

For many students with disabilities, eating is work and should be made as easy as possible. The work of eating can be minimized in many ways. First, increase the student's focus on the meal. This might involve moving to a special area of the room with fewer distractions. In most cases, students with feeding difficulties eat better in one-on-one situations or in small groups with few distractions. Second, include foods that are easier for the student to control both manually and intra-orally. For example, foods with smooth textures such as pudding and applesauce are much easier for a student to handle than soup or pizza. These foods require a much higher level of oral-motor abilities. A variety of adaptive utensils are available to facilitate independence and optimal oral-motor function during mealtime. Examples include spoons with built-up or curved handles, specialized cups and bowls with higher sides that will not shift on the table, and cups with lids and straws to promote the student's ability to suck (Figure 4).

Feeding Students with Sensory Processing Delays

Children with sensory processing problems often exhibit oral-motor/feeding delays. These children often present with sensory defensiveness in their bodies as well as in and around their mouths. They demonstrate aversive responses to touch of their arms, legs, and hands, as well as in and around their mouths. They cannot tolerate certain tastes, textures, or temperatures in their mouths.

Treatment involves a whole-body approach, not just an oral-motor approach. Brushing techniques as described in the sensory processing portion of this book can be the first approach. The COTA can then begin gradually to introduce a variety of tactile experiences to the child's hands, legs, body, and facial area. The COTA should never force a tactile experience on a child. If a child is showing a negative response, the COTA might need to try a new experience. An oral stimulation program can be initiated. It is recommended that the COTA wear protective gloves when working with saliva. Use firm wiping/rubbing of the face, gradually incorporating the cheeks and lips as tolerated. The COTA might want to use a NUK® brush to provide firm input to the biting surfaces (teeth). The NUK brush can be incorporated for tactile stimulation to the inner cheeks, gums, and tongue, if the student tolerates this. Remember never to force oral stimulation on a child. The COTA may introduce a small vibrator or vibrating toy and allow this input to the outer and inner oral cavity. Allow the child to control this input if he has the motor skills to do so. When introducing food to students with sensory processing delays, try a variety of textures, tastes, and temperatures. A particular texture could cause extreme irritation in a child; therefore, a gradual approach to increasing a new texture generally helps.

Feeding Students with Low Muscle Tone

Children with generalized low muscle tone usually have some degree of oral-motor/feeding delay. Increasing their overall muscle tone as well as their oral musculature tone is recommended. Bouncing them on a ball or a lap is a good first step. To increase tone in the facial area, the COTA can do some facial play with the child. Play pat-a-cake, peek-a-boo, and other children's games that incorporate patting, tapping, stroking, and other types of tactile and proprioceptive stimulation of the cheeks and lips (Morris & Klein, 1987). A vibrating toy to the mouth also will help increase muscle activity around the mouth. Often, children with low muscle tone drool and posture their tongues out of their mouths. Drooling often occurs as a result of poor oral-motor control, a decrease in the frequency of spontaneous swallow, and/or a reduction in the sensory awareness necessary for swallowing (Johnson & Scott, 1993). It is advisable to vary temperature, taste, pressure, and the texture of food and objects in the mouth to increase general sensory awareness and discrimination (Morris & Klein, 1987). This approach should help to decrease some of the drooling. Talk with the child about the concept of wet and dry, and provide her with a verbal reminder to swallow. With some children, gum chewing will help to decrease the drooling, as this keeps their oral musculature active. The OTR and COTA need to decide whether this is an appropriate technique and educate the teacher about gum chewing. To increase active use of the tongue, encourage food to be licked from specific sites, using the tongue only. Place the food (i.e., jam, honey) at various sites inside the mouth, as well as on and around the lips (Johnson & Scott, 1993). Or, try having the student lick envelopes, stickers, or lollipops. This also should help increase tongue activity. Providing firm downward pressure on the tongue during feeding should help to inhibit the tongue-out-of-mouth posture. The COTA can encourage many oral-motor resistive activities such as blowing bubbles and drinking thickened liquids from a straw to help improve the child's oral strength.

Feeding Students with Hypertonicity (i.e., CP)

Children with increased muscle tone and extensor patterns have limited oral-motor/feeding abilities and often exhibit jaw thrusting, a tonic bite reflex, and abnormal patterning of the tongue, lip, and jaw. The key to treatment is first to ensure proper positioning as discussed earlier. The COTA might need to use jaw-stability techniques to help the child experience a closed-mouth sensation and educate the teacher in this particular technique (Figure 3). An oral stimulation program should be implemented because children with increased muscle tone often have oral defensiveness and a tonic bite reflex. The tonic bite reflex occurs when the jaw moves upward into a tightly clenched posture while the teeth are stimulated by a finger, spoon, or other object, making it difficult for the child to open the mouth (Morris & Klein, 1987). Plastic cafeteria spoons or forks

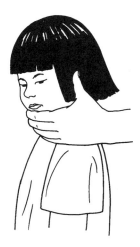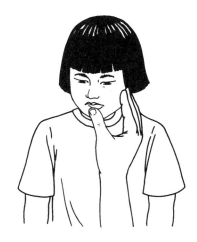

Figure 3. The COTA can use jaw-stability techniques such as these to help the child experience a closed-mouth sensation.

should never be used to feed a student with a tonic bite reflex, as he might bite the utensil and break it off in his mouth, causing potentially dangerous choking. When working with a student with a tonic bite reflex, the COTA should not pull the spoon back, as this will make the child clench harder. Try applying deep, firm pressure down through the biting surfaces (teeth) and the student should release the bite. The student needs to be introduced to a good oral-stimulation program in an attempt to eliminate this reflex. When feeding the student with a tonic bite, the COTA should present the spoon or cup on the lower lip, not the teeth. When the child initiates a suckle/swallow from the closed-mouth position, the tonic bite reflex is not as strong. To inhibit abnormal patterning of the tongue, lip, and jaw, the COTA must first try to normalize the tone in the whole body and then position the student appropriately. If the student uses a tongue-thrust pattern, try to change the consistency of the food so that tongue protrusion is not needed to move the food backward. Use jaw-stability techniques to help maintain the tongue in the mouth (Figure 3). Students with increased muscle tone generally benefit from the use of adaptive utensils to promote some level of success or independence. Following are some examples of the many adaptive feeding devices available (Figure 4).

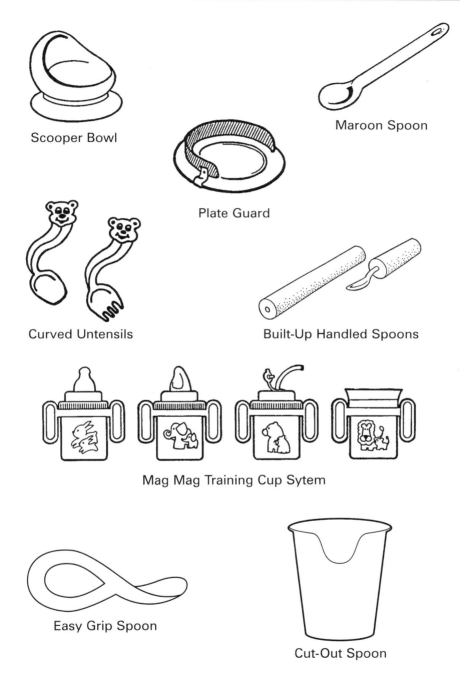

Scooper Bowl

Plate Guard

Maroon Spoon

Curved Untensils

Built-Up Handled Spoons

Mag Mag Training Cup Sytem

Easy Grip Spoon

Cut-Out Spoon

Figure 4. Students with increased muscle tone have many adaptive feeding devices available to assist them.

Fine-Motor Control

Fine-motor control is the ability to utilize one's hands and fingers precisely in a skilled activity (Bissell, et al., 1988). A child needs a solid sensory and motor foundation to demonstrate good fine-motor skills. For good fine-motor abilities, a student must have good muscle and joint stability, especially in the neck, trunk, and upper extremities. The eye muscles must work in a coordinated manner to track objects in the environment and guide the hand in function. A subconscious awareness of how the fingers and hands move in space also is important for good fine-motor skills. Good tactile discrimination and appropriate hand strength help the student control tools. The ability to judge the visual-spacial relationship of objects accurately is essential for the precision required in fine-motor control (Bissell, et al., 1988). Motor planning and coordination between the two sides of the body are important for fine-motor coordination and the development of a specific hand dominance. Hand skills develop and lead to a student's ability to control tools such as scissors and pencils.

There is a developmental sequence to learning hand skills just as there is a developmental sequence to achieving gross-motor milestones.

Initially, the whole hand is used to grasp an object. The gross-release ability follows the ability to gross grasp. Initially, release is crude and random. The child gains better control of release through play as she grasps and releases many toys. Activities to help increase release skills include stacking blocks, placing items into a container, and tossing beanbags or balls.

Fine grasp is used when a child is able to control each finger independently in relation to the thumb. Examples include poking with the index finger, pointing with the index finger, and picking up small objects. Skill and dexterity in using refined grasp patterns is achieved as the child finger feeds and plays with pegs, beads, and crayons. A child develops a raking grasp, a radial raking grasp, an inferior pincer, and finally, a neat pincer grasp.

Tool control requires coordinated use of the hands. A student goes through a developmental sequence for holding a writing utensil. Initially, the student uses a palmar-supinate (or gross-palmar) grasp and then advances to a digital-pronate (or pronated) grasp, then a static tripod, and finally, a mature dynamic tripod grasp (Figure 5). Writing is considered a high-level, fine-motor task, and the student must have all the preliminary fine-motor abilities to control a pencil successfully in order to write effectively.

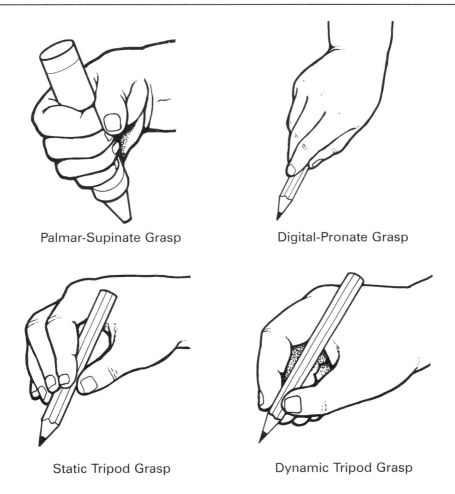

Palmar-Supinate Grasp

Digital-Pronate Grasp

Static Tripod Grasp

Dynamic Tripod Grasp

Figure 5. Students go through a four-step developmental sequence to learn the fine-motor task of using a writing utensil.*

Typical classroom activities that involve hand skills include using tools (pencils, scissors, other utensils); using two hands together (one to hold, the other to manipulate); managing book bags; manipulating door knobs; and exercising other activities that are a regular part of the child's education. The development of dexterous hand skills depends on the interaction of all joints in the upper extremity—the scapulothoracic, glenohumeral,

*Illustrations from *The Erhardt Developmental Prehension Assessment,* copyright © 1994 by Rhoda P. Erhardt. Published by Therapy Skill Builders, a division of The Psychological Corporation, San Antonio, Texas 78204-2498, USA, (800) 228-0752. Reprinted by permission.

elbow, and wrist (Benbow, 1998). In addition to adequate range of motion, every proximal joint must provide a stable base of support for the joint distal. When treatment is provided to improve hand skills (fine-motor skill development), other factors to be considered are positioning of the child, inhibition or facilitation of tone, and postural control.

The development of fine-motor skills facilitates skills such as manipulating fasteners, writing, and using scissors (Usman & Szkut, 1993). Using a hole puncher and pushing pegs into clay are two enjoyable activities that increase finger strength and control. Activities to develop grip and pinch strength include any that involve pinching and gripping against resistance. For example, pulling pop beads apart, using toy construction sets and squeeze toys, playing with grip-handle squirt guns, and squeezing sponges in a water table all involve pinching and gripping against resistance.

To enhance the development of the child's web space (the circle formed by the index finger and thumb), which is needed to hold a pencil correctly, a variety of activities are suggested. These activities include popping the plastic bubbles on packing sheets, opening and closing bags that seal, winding up wind-up toys that have a knob, and using an eye dropper to make pictures by mixing food coloring with water and dripping it onto paper towels.

Activities to improve a student's fine-motor control and isolated finger movements include: (1) rolling $1/4$-inch to $1/8$-inch balls of clay or play dough between the tip of the thumb and the tips of the index and middle fingers; (2) picking up small objects with tweezers and assorted tongs; and (3) twisting open a small tube of toothpaste. To facilitate development of the skill fingers (thumb, index, and middle fingers), which are necessary for the refinement of handwriting and scissors skills, use a spray bottle to squirt water onto a picture and cut strips of paper, straws, or rolls of clay.

Students with poor handwriting frequently exhibit poor proximal stability (Amundson, 1992). To encourage co-contraction through the neck, shoulders, elbows, and wrists, students can imitate certain animal walks such as the crab walk, the bear walk, and the inchworm creep. Older children might prefer push-ups on the floor or against the wall, or resistive exercises that incorporate Thera-Band® or elastic tubing. Cleaning chalkboards and table tops or pushing open heavy external doors are good functional activities in the school setting that naturally promote stability.

Activities that involve tactile awareness to reinforce writing skills include drawing lines and copying shapes using shaving cream, sand, or finger paints, and completing simple dot-to-dot pictures and mazes. Coloring and scissors activities are excellent for developing a smooth, graded movement of the arm and hand.

Other factors to consider are sitting posture (desktop and chair at suitable heights to allow the child to sit with feet flat on the floor), writing tools (pencil grips, shapes and sizes of pencils), paper position, pencil grasp, and writing surfaces. Working on a vertical or inclined surface helps the child develop the shoulder and wrist strength essential for writing. This can be done by writing on a blackboard, an easel, paper taped on the wall, or by using an inclined writing board (Figure 6).

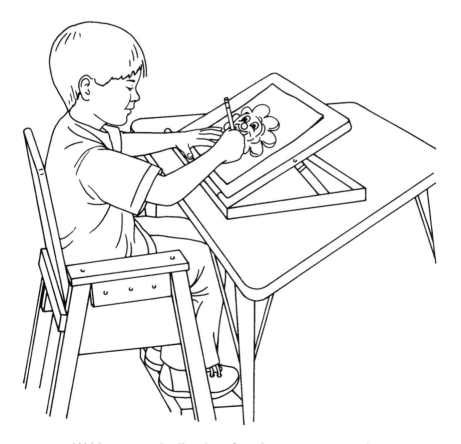

Figure 6. Writing on an inclined surface is one way a student can develop the shoulder and wrist strength essential for writing.

Playing selected children's games is another excellent way to improve fine-motor control. Some of the games that increase the development of fine-motor skills are Trouble®, Bed Bugs, Crocodile Dentist, Connect Four®, Lite Brite, and Magna Doodle. By using games that involve spatial con-struction, such as Legos®, Tinkertoys®, building blocks, and origami, the child develops both fine-motor control and motor planning.

Many fine-motor treatment activities work on several components of fine-motor development. For example, pop beads help with hand strength, bilateral coordination, and finger isolation and dexterity. Because of this, the COTA is able to use the same toy to work on different skills depending on how he engages the child to use the toy. During a particular activity, it is very important that the COTA be familiar with the student's goal. The fine-motor activities are endless and the COTA can be very creative in achieving the underlying goal while the student is simply *playing*!

Sensory-Motor Treatment

OTRs and COTAs often treat children with sensory processing disorders. Sensory processing diagnoses might include autism, pervasive developmental disorder (PDD), learning disabled (LD), attention deficit disorder (ADD), attention deficit/hyperactive disorder (ADHD), and behavioral dysfunction. In general, children who have difficulty using and processing tactile, proprioceptive, and vestibular input could benefit from sensory-motor treatment. If a sensory-motor problem exists, a COTA can offer suggestions on how to adapt the environment and assist the child in modifying her responses to the environmental stimulation (Koomar, 1990). There are many different types of sensory processing problems. They include tactile defensiveness, gravitational insecurity, motor-planning delays, auditory defensiveness, an underactive vestibular system, oral defensiveness, and poor balance-coordination skills (clumsiness). The next section will provide general treatment suggestions for children with sensory delays.

Tactile

Tactile defensiveness is a common sensory problem. Students may resist being touched by other children, touching certain textures with their own hands, or even feel irritated by the clothing that touches their bodies.

One approach to implement for students with tactile defensiveness is a brushing program developed by Patricia Wilbarger and Julia Wilbarger, who are OTRs with extensive training and experience in the area of sensory defensiveness. The COTA should be taught this specific technique by the supervising OTR. The technique involves using a corn brush to brush the child's skin. This includes brushing the arms, back, legs, feet, and hands with a pressure-touch sensation to quickly fire up multiple pressure-touch receptors in a large area (Figure 7). The brushing is then followed by a compression component. Deep compression is given to the key joints of the upper and lower extremities. The COTA also should be taught compression techniques by the supervising OTR, as there are precautions and specific procedures that must be followed. This brushing technique can be used when there is evidence of sensory defensiveness. To enhance carryover in the classroom, teachers can learn this brushing technique from a COTA or OTR.

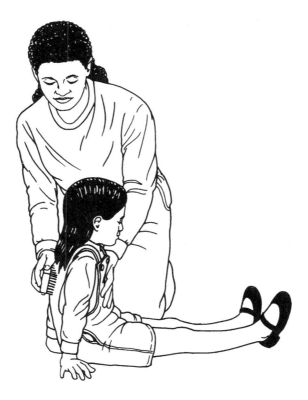

Figure 7. This brushing technique followed by the application of deep pressure to the upper and lower extremities helps students with tactile defensiveness.

There are a variety of tactile activities available to children with tactile defensiveness, such as engaging play with the child in a shaving cream activity or picking art toys from a bin filled with a sensory medium such as rice or macaroni. Some children with tactile problems benefit from having a Koosh Ball® or other tactile toy at their desk to hold and manipulate. The ball bath, which is a large pool filled with many bright colored balls, provides a nice activity for tactile input throughout the entire body (Figure 8). Often found at fast-food restaurants or children's play centers, ball baths offer a child the opportunity to submerge his body in the balls.

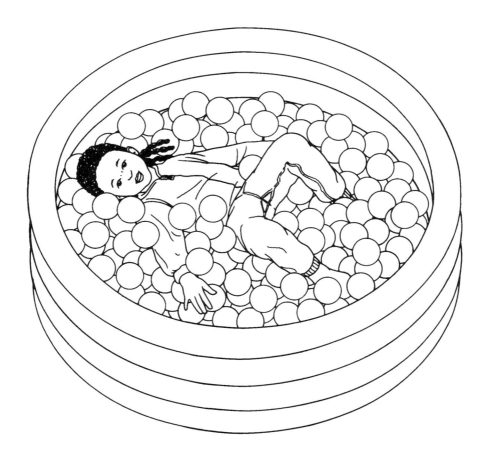

Figure 8.   A ball bath provides the opportunity for tactile input throughout the body.

Proprioceptive

Many children with sensory processing disorders need strong propriocep-tive input. To provide proprioceptive input, the therapist needs equipment that can be used to provide resistance to the muscles (Koomar, 1990). Each child has individual needs for proprioception based on his or her unique sensory system. COTAs need to grade the proprioceptive activity based on the individual student's needs.

Below is a general list of activities that provide the student with proprio-ceptive input:

- Bouncing on a therapy ball

- Wearing a weighted vest

- Jumping on a mini-trampoline

- Giving a student firm bear hugs

- Wrapping a child tightly in a blanket

- Eating resistive foods (gum, licorice, fruit roll-ups)

- Pulling one's self on a scooter

- Kneeling or lying on the stomach to do an activity typically done at a desktop

Heavy work is a form of proprioception that requires exertion on the student's part. Heavy work activities that can be incorporated into the classroom include:

- Pushing desks/carts

- Carrying heavy objects

- Holding doors open

- Stacking/lifting boxes

- Cleaning and wiping chalkboards

- Pulling the other students in a wagon

Vestibular

To provide vestibular input effectively, COTAs need to have equipment that can provide input in all planes of movement at a variety of speeds and in an angular as well as a linear manner (Koomar, 1990). Vestibular input is very powerful. Whenever possible, the student should be allowed to control the amount of input she receives by providing the input to herself. Vestibular input can be provided by the COTA's use of any of the suspended equipment and swings commonly found in occupational therapy departments. The COTA can change the speed or direction of this equipment to offer the specific type of input needed by a particular student. The swing can provide inhibitory vestibular input if the COTA uses slow, rhythmical, and linear motions, or it can give more excitatory/stimulatory input if the movement of the swing is fast, irregular, and unpredictable. Below is a list of other activities that can provide students with vestibular input:

- Riding a scooter board down a ramp
- Riding a bicycle or tricycle
- Bouncing on a Hippity-Hop
- Moving a therapy ball
- Sitting on a movable seat cushion at a desk
- Allowing movement breaks periodically throughout the day
- Riding a Sit-n-Spin

Visual/Olfactory/Gustatory/Auditory

When looking at the sensory systems, one also must consider the visual, olfactory, gustatory (taste), and auditory. A student will not be able to perform in the classroom if he has sensory processing problems.

Seating placement of a student can be critical to her success in the classroom. A COTA needs to consider the lighting and activity level for a student who cannot tolerate a lot of visual input. Brighter or dimmer lighting can enable a student to function better. A particular student might need to sit near or far away from the window depending on his visual sensitivity. Some children need a high-contrast background for reading and writing activities. Others need to sit near or far away from the high-traffic aisle in the classroom depending on the noise level. Some students cannot tolerate the sounds common to a classroom and may need to wear headphones that provide musical input.

A food smell might be too noxious for yet another student to focus, if she is seated near the lunchroom. Some students require particular tastes (candy/gum) in their mouth to stay alert while doing academic work. The list of things that can disturb a child with sensory processing problems can go on and on. The main idea is to remember that each student may have unique sensory needs. The OTR/COTA team can help ensure that the sensory needs of each student are being met.

Motor Planning

Motor planning is the brain's ability to conceive, organize, and carry out a sequence of unfamiliar actions. Motor planning is the first step in learning a new skill. Good motor-planning abilities require accurate information from all sensory systems of the body. Motor planning will be compromised if any of the sensory processing is impaired. A child with poor motor planning may seem clumsy, accident prone, and messy. Motor-planning abilities are challenged in the classroom every time a child is presented with a new assignment or a variation of a familiar motor task. A child with motor-planning problems may have difficulty finishing work on time, as he has no idea how to start or finish a task. Another child with motor-planning delays may rush through a task without being able to recognize the steps of the task as they relate to the end product. This child typically will turn in messy work. Motor planning is developed when a child experiments with how parts relate to the whole, as with toys such as puzzles, take-apart toys, or models. Games such as patty-cake, peekaboo, Simon says, and follow the leader require motor-planning abilities. Other activities to help a child with motor-planning problems include:

- Obstacle courses—student maneuvers a scooter board around cones
- Getting on/off a variety of playground equipment
- Jumping jacks
- Any new sporting task

Bilateral Coordination

The ability to coordinate the left and right sides of the body and cross midline is an indication that both sides of the brain can work well together. The development of gross- and fine-motor skills relies on coordination of the two sides of the body. Bilateral coordination is essential to participating in writing and cutting activities. A student with poor bilateral coordination will adjust his body to avoid crossing the body's midline, frequently will switch hands during fine-motor tasks, and have great difficulty developing a hand dominance. The student may be unable to coordinate the movement of one hand while using the other hand to stabilize. Below is a list of bilateral (two-handed) activities:

- Stringing beads/pop beads

- Cutting with scissors

- Jumping rope

- Jumping jacks

- Pouring and dumping activities

- Writing and holding the paper with the non-dominant hand

- Riding and steering a bicycle

- Participating in a football passing game

- Clapping during imitation games

- Climbing a ladder

- Playing on playground equipment such as the monkey bars

- Participating in scooter board activities

Following are activities to promote crossing the midline:

- Placing the toys/paper to one side so that the student will cross the middle to play with them

- Playing Simon says

- Playing wire-bead games

- Drawing lines to connect dots on a chalkboard

- Reading while using a finger to follow words across a page

- Writing activities

- Doing aerobics

- Sporting activities, such as swinging a bat or playing tennis, Ping-Pong, golf, or a similar activity

Body Awareness

Awareness of the body comes from input from the muscles and joints. Receptors in the joints and muscles tell the brain how the joints are being moved. This information lets the brain know where each part is and how it is moving through space. A student with poor body awareness may have problems knowing where his body is in relation to objects. The student may fall out of his chair frequently or have difficulty getting dressed or getting into or out of the bus. This student may press too hard or too softly on a pencil, as he cannot grade the pressure. Frequently, students with body-awareness problems appear sloppy and clumsy, and have disorganized personal belongings. Ideas to promote increased body awareness include:

- Using a mirror during movement activities so that the student can see where her extremities are

- Crawling, climbing, lifting, and carrying heavy objects

- Pulling and pushing toys that offer resistance

- Using weighted beanbags to play tossing games

- Providing firm pressure through the shoulders during an activity

Many students with motor-planning/sensory deficits are labeled as having behavioral problems when, in truth, a sensory deficit is the cause of their actions. The OTR/COTA team can help identify these students and offer assistance.

Sensory Stimulation for Students With Profound Disabilities

Children learn about their bodies and environment by interacting with their environment and by sensory input. A child who is unable to move or use her hands has difficulty initiating play or interactions designed to give sensory input. Information gathered through the senses is the basis for learning. Students with profound cognitive or physical disabilities have limited sensory awareness and therefore need assistance in tuning in to their senses. COTAs can offer a multisensory approach to meet the individual needs of the student with profound disabilities through sensory stimulation. Service delivery can be direct treatment and consultation with the teacher to adapt the group activity for the individual student. An example of direct treatment might be to apply lotion with a sponge or massage the student's arms, face, or hands. An example of a consultation might include showing the teacher how to mix sand in paint to vary the texture during a group painting activity.

Active stimulation is encouraged whenever possible because it more likely will engage the child's inner drive and lead to more complex adaptive responses (Clark, Mailloux, & Parham, 1985). Passive sensory stimulation, however, may need to be used with students with profound involvement who appear to have difficulty processing sensory information.

The vestibular system responds to movement and gravity. It helps a child use his eyes and hands to work together, and it also enables him to learn about his position in space. Movement activities for a student with profound involvement might include being swung in an adaptive swing, moved over uneven surfaces while in a wheelchair, bounced on a ball, or rocked in a rocking chair.

Tactile (touch) input is received by the receptors in the skin. While firm deep pressure is organizing and calming, light touch is alerting and can be unsettling. Because of this, hand-over-hand assistance to manipulate classroom materials may be necessary. Texture tables or boards using textures that range from the rough and course to the soft and smooth can be introduced throughout the day while the student is positioned in a wheelchair or other piece of adaptive equipment.

Visual stimulation also increases awareness of the environment. Many students are visual learners. A few classroom activities that promote visual stimulation are bright colored mobiles, games that promote visual tracking, and playing in front of mirrors.

Auditory stimulation such as listening to music or mimicking sounds also is important in a good sensory-stimulation program.

Last of all, the sense of smell can trigger a perception or provide a clue or memory for a concept that we wish to stress. Scent can be added to clay or paint. Make smelling objects part of your activity. For example, if the classroom activity involves fruit, encourage the students to smell it.

When using a multisensory stimulation approach, you must watch the student carefully and monitor his body language, speech, or other communication styles to gauge his reaction to the stimulation. Then you will need to adjust your activities accordingly.

Assistive Technology

The 1997 reauthorization of the Individuals with Disabilities Act (IDEA) mandated that every IEP team examine the child's need for assistive technology, which is defined as any item, piece of equipment, or product system (whether it is acquired commercially or modified or customized) that is used to increase, maintain, or improve the functional capabilities of a child with a disability (Reed, 1998). Assistive technology is anything that can help a person with a disability do something that she otherwise cannot do or that helps her do it better (Reed, 1998). It can be an extension on a light switch that enables a child in a wheelchair to turn on a light, a wheelchair, or a pencil grip that helps a child grasp a pencil. Assistive technology is most appropriate when a child wants to complete a task but is unsuccessful because of a physical or sensory limitation (Reed, 1998), and it is available for spoken and written communication, mobility, seeing, reading, eating, feeding, hearing, dressing, and playing (Figure 9). It also is necessary when remediation and environmental modifications are not enough to enable the student to function optimally in the classroom.

Other examples of assistive technology commonly used in the schools are switches and switch-activated devices. A switch is a mechanical device that closes an electrical circuit to turn things on and off. Switches are housed in different ways to enable students with different abilities to access them. They can be used to operate everything from computers, communication devices, environmental control systems, and mobility aids to the simplest toys and appliances, many of which already are switch-adapted. Any toy that is battery-operated can be used with a switch. An interrupter cable must be used with these toys to enable them to work with a switch. The copper end of the adaptor cable is inserted into the battery compartment on top of the battery. The end where the jack is located is then plugged into the switch.

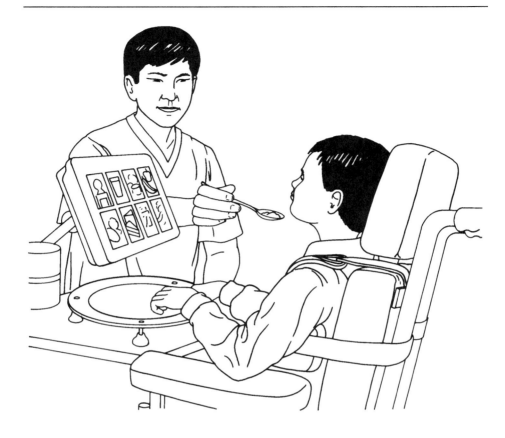

Figure 9. A student expresses his food choice using an augmentative communication device while positioned in a wheelchair.

For the computer, alternative keyboards such as IntelliKeys® with magnetic-coded overlays and TouchWindows™ with specialized software are available. The IntelliKeys keyboard provides physical, visual, and cognitive access for students with a wide range of disabilities. The keyboard features large, well-spaced keys and high-contrast colors to make it easy for students to locate letters or numbers. A student with limited motor skills often can successfully interact with the computer using Intellikeys. When using a TouchWindow, all the student needs to do is touch the computer screen to control the computer. Also, there are alternative pointing devices such as the trackball, touch pad, and head pointer as well as specialized on-screen keyboards such as the WiVik 2 or Discovery screen that provide a student with disabilities with an alternative to the standard keyboard-activated computer use.

Use of Specialized Equipment in Therapy

A variety of specialized equipment can be used in therapy—bolsters, balls, mini-trampolines, scooters, and swings—and positioning equipment such as standers, corner seats, wedges, feeder seats, sidelyers, bolster chairs, and wheelchairs.

Bolsters

Unlike balls, bolsters limit movement to one plane of motion, enabling the COTA to work on single components of movement. When using bolsters, always be sure that the student's weight-bearing hip stays centered on top of the bolster. If you want the hip to be the point of stability for the balance reaction, you must make sure that the bolster is large enough to prevent the student's foot from touching the floor; otherwise, the foot on the floor becomes the point of stability.

While sitting on a bolster, the student responds to passive weight shifts laterally. When straddling the bolster anteriorly or posteriorly while sitting on the end with the legs in front, she can weight shift actively while reaching laterally, anteriorly, and posteriorly with rotation. If the student sits on a bolster that's tilted on an incline, this increases anterior pelvic tilt and elongates the trunk. The student can work on transitions as he straddles the bolster and moves from sitting to standing while reaching forward for an object.

Standing on a bolster can strengthen or stretch ankle plantarflexors as well as improve trunk control and balance reactions.

In prone, the student can straddle a bolster and work on quadruped weight bearing. Trunk extension can be achieved in prone with the bolster positioned at the hips.

The bolster can be suspended from the ceiling and moved to provide vestibular stimulation, including vertical stimulation, linear acceleration, and head-righting reactions (Figure 10).

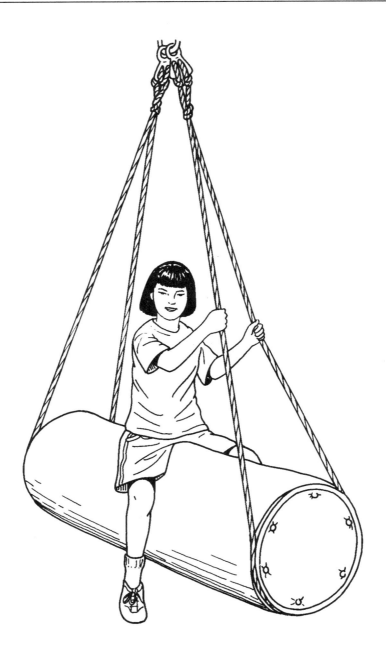

Figure 10. One of the many ways that a student can use a bolster.

Therapy Balls

Therapy balls can be used to facilitate balance reactions in the anterior, posterior, lateral, and diagonal planes of movement, but they are more difficult surfaces to control than bolsters. The size of the ball depends on the student's size, the size of the room available, and the goals to be achieved. If the student is very small or severely involved, it is easier to work on a large ball because it has a larger surface area, although it is more difficult for the COTA to control balls larger than the student.

The inflation level of the ball depends on the COTA's preference and the goals of the therapy session. A ball that is not fully inflated is preferable because, as the student sits on the ball, the bottom flattens and provides a larger surface area that prevents the ball from rolling away. Sometimes, a firmly inflated ball, which moves more quickly, is indicated.

Ball techniques used in prone can focus on many areas including elongating the rectus abdominus, lengthening the latissimus, promoting thoracic extension, improving joint mobility, and strengthening. The student can lie prone on the ball and be rolled anteriorly, posteriorly, or laterally to elicit protective and righting reactions. The student can prop herself on the elbows to work on cervical spine extension or weight bearing through the shoulders. Supine to sidelying transitions and rolling supine to prone are other positions easily facilitated on the ball. While working on weight shifting, the COTA can facilitate a variety of responses, including unilateral, bilateral, and diagonal control depending on the student's ability and the stability of the ball.

In sitting, anterior and posterior weight shifting facilitates pelvic mobility, and lateral weight shifting facilitates lateral balance reactions. Sitting is an excellent position in which to work on lengthening many trunk, pelvic, and lower extremity muscles. In addition, transitions from prone to sitting or from sitting to sidelying can be facilitated (Figure 11).

Kneeling on the ball or using it in front of the body as a support requires joint alignment between the pelvis and spine, and the pelvis and femurs. Transitions from quadruped to kneeling or from kneeling to half-kneeling also can be facilitated.

Therapy involving standing on the ball is an excellent way to challenge balance and promote weight shifting. The student can stand on a small ball with one foot, stand on top of the ball with two feet, or stand with the ball in front of the body and use it as a support. Activities for rotation between the upper and lower body using a small ball can include passing the ball under the student's legs, over the student's head, and to the side. Other techniques include standing and catching a ball that is passed in a variety of ways and carrying the ball in front, which promotes trunk extension.

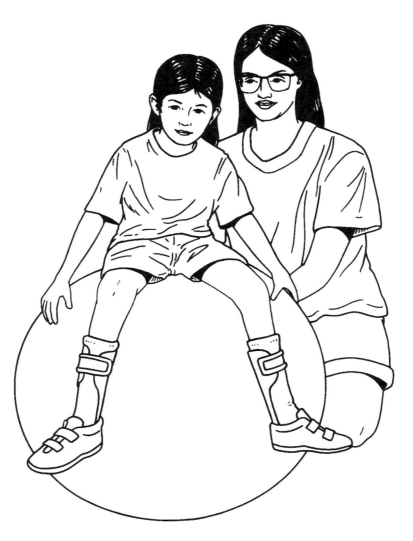

Figure 11. Weight shifting to facilitate balance reactions while on the ball.

The therapy ball is an excellent tool to use for vestibular and proprioceptive input. Bouncing a child on the ball provides this type of input. It can be rhythmical to help calm the student or fast and irregular to alert the student. Rolling the ball over the student (*sandwich games*) is a great form of proprioceptive input. The student needs to be an active participant in the ball activities and not a passive recipient of the stimulation.

Mini-trampoline

The mini-trampoline is an excellent form of joint compression and proprioceptive input for a student with sensory-motor delays. The COTA may incorporate using a weighted vest while the student is jumping on the trampoline to provide even greater input. Many students with sensory processing difficulties need this proprioceptive input repeatedly throughout the day. Once they receive it, they can return to a desk activity in the classroom and focus on their work again.

Swings/Suspended Equipment

Swings are basic therapeutic tools for promoting vestibular sensory stimulation in a variety of positions. Suspended equipment is essential for the COTA to provide vestibular stimulation (Figure 12). Swinging equipment will provide rotary, vertical, and horizontal linear movement. Some good sources of vestibular stimulation are the bolster, tire, and platform swings; the net hammock; and the frog swing, which provides a natural combination of proprioceptive input and linear-vestibular input. It enables the student to bounce on his hands and feet while being supported on his stomach in the sling. The child can be in direct control of the amount of stimulation he receives.

The suspension system needs to be securely supported for safety. The use of steel beams of the building structure, along with eyebolts, suspended chains, and hooks is important. A variety of suspended equipment structures are available to allow for more portable use. Southpaw Enterprises Inc. sells suspension systems and hardware as well as many of the suspended equipment items. Please refer to specific resources when installing a suspension system.

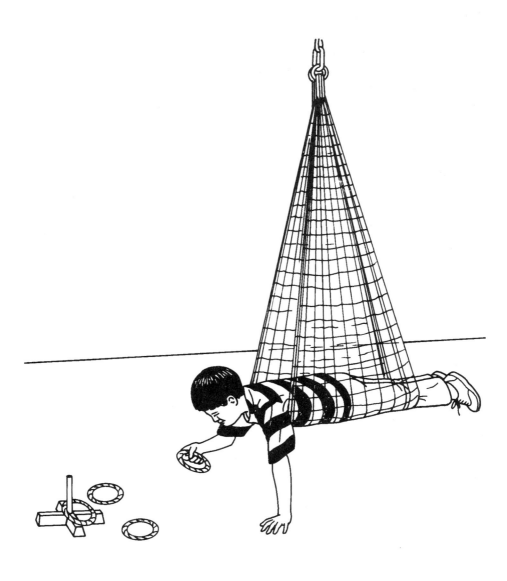

Figure 12. This student plays a ring-toss game while suspended in a net swing.

Scooters

Scooters are used to develop neck, shoulder, and arm muscles as well as to encourage movement, balance reactions, and directionality. In supine, students can practice leg strengthening by pushing their legs off a wall. While in prone, students can propel a scooter using their arms or both their arms and legs, thus promoting crawling. Students also can hold onto a rope using their upper extremities while crawling up the rope. This activity promotes head and upper back-extension strength against gravity. In sitting, the students can practice balance as the COTA pulls them around by a rope that they hold onto.

An excellent way to work on trunk stability, especially in students with hypotonicity, is for the COTA to sit on a scooter and have the student push her down the hall. Another therapy idea is to have the COTA sit on the scooter and have the student pull her around by a rope. This enables the student to work on backward walking or forward walking while promoting trunk stability and strength.

Scooter boards can be used to ride down a ramp to provide linear-vestibular stimulation (Figure 13). The COTA may incorporate spinning on the scooter board if appropriate for the student. Heavy work or deep proprioceptive input can be achieved through pulling and pushing one's self or others on the scooter. Having the student pull himself up a ramp using a rope or the edge of the ramp is an effective form of deep proprioception. The student can descend the ramp in prone to promote use of the extensors and then crash into building blocks to get added proprioceptive input. The activities are endless, and the COTA can use her creativity to promote this type of sensory input.

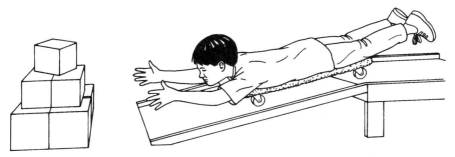

Figure 13. A student is receiving linear-vestibular and proprioceptive input by descending the ramp and crashing.

Positioning/Adaptive Equipment

An important role for the COTA is one of providing and fabricating adaptive equipment needed by the child to function in the classroom—equipment needed for sitting, as well as standers, corner chairs, bolster chairs, and sidelyers. This also includes adaptive equipment for managing classroom materials, writing, eating, dressing, and toileting. Much of the equipment for managing the classroom environment already has been discussed. This section will focus on positioning equipment for the student with disabilities.

Many students in special education require the use of a variety of positioning devices to assist in the educational process. Positioning always should be done for a specific activity. In other words, the position is not an end in itself; it is a means for the student to participate effectively in an activity or educational goal. Positioning devices or adaptive equipment can be useful in controlling abnormal movement responses. Equipment that aligns the student's body correctly can assist in preventing or decreasing the severity of many deformities. Abnormal muscle tone can lead to deformities of the bones and muscles. These muscles that pull body parts in the same abnormal patterns of movement can actually change the structure of the bones and muscles permanently, requiring surgical correction. Examples of this include dislocated hips, scoliosis of the spine, and tightening of the ankle tendons.

The two important principles to remember when positioning students are symmetry and normal postural alignment of the body. Symmetry means that both sides of the body are the same and the head is in the middle of the body (midline). Because abnormal muscle tone can pull the body into asymmetrical postures, equipment is helpful to maintain symmetry. Alignment refers to positioning the body in a straight line. Proper alignment includes a straight back without curvature, weight distributed equally over the hips, feet placed directly under the knees, and the toes pointed straight ahead.

Often, students with abnormal muscle tone cannot achieve perfect symmetry and alignment; therefore, every attempt should be made to achieve the best possible position.

Proper positioning can promote more proximal stability, resulting in controlled fine-motor movements or more successful attempts at movement. It can also facilitate better feeding and swallowing. The student who is properly positioned should have improved access to his environment.

The effect of positioning on verbal and nonverbal communication should not be underestimated. Proper positioning aids communication in several ways. For sound production, the student must be aligned to allow for a good breathing pattern. If the student uses a communication device, proper positioning assists in the upper-extremity or head movement needed to activate the communication device.

Standers

Prone, supine, and vertical standers enable the student to be upright and experience the sensation of weight bearing. The standing position is especially important for older students because it is socially beneficial for them to view their surroundings from an age-appropriate height (Figure 14).

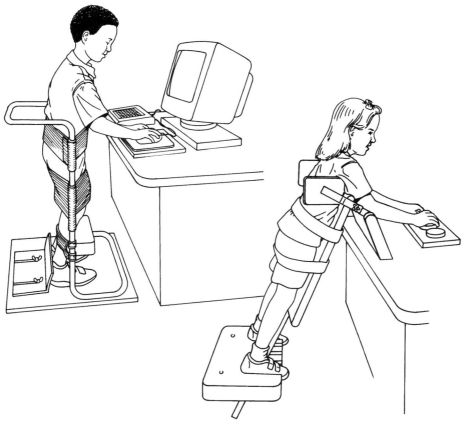

Figure 14. One student (left) uses a vertical stander while playing a game on the computer, and another student operates switches while using a prone stander.

Bolster chairs

Bolster chairs are most appropriate for students with hypertonicity or with fluctuating tone (athetosis). These students need a wide base of support and hip flexion with abduction to achieve their best pelvic alignment for sitting. Bolster chairs with lateral pelvic supports, a firm back, and foot supports aid symmetry and alignment without the necessity of restraints. These chairs are an excellent seating alternative for children who *W-sit*—with their legs in knee flexion and internally rotated. Prolonged sitting in a *W* position may lead to tightness in the internal rotators and adductors of the hip and limit the student's ability to move into and out of sitting. Bolster chairs maintain hip flexion and adduction with external rotation, a position that promotes movement in sitting.

Feeder seats

Feeder seats, also known as floor sitters, offer students good alignment for feeding, operating a switch, or playing upright with toys. They provide lateral support and have an adductor wedge built into the seat to discourage excessive adduction and promote good hip and knee alignment. These seats also can be placed inside a net swing to offer vestibular sensory stimulation even to the most severely involved student.

Corner seats

For students who are unable to sit independently, corner seats provide the opportunity to sit upright without assistance. Tri-wall, a thick corrugated cardboard, can be used for fabricating adaptive seating devices such as corner seats. While sitting in a corner seat, the student can engage in many upright activities such as an art project, listening to a story, or operating a switch (Figure 15).

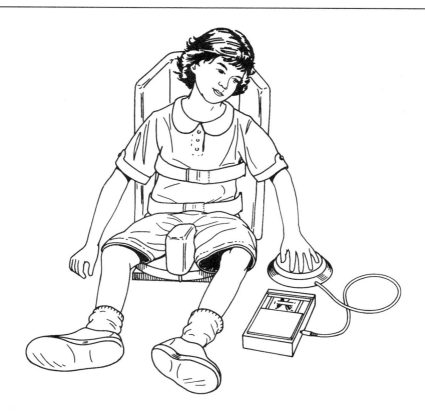

This student uses a switch to listen to music while
Figure 15. sitting in a corner chair.

Sidelyers

Sidelyers often are used with students who require alternatives to prone or supine positioning. Sidelyers are used to attain symmetry and make it easier for the hands to function at the middle of the body. In sidelying, the effect of abnormal reflexes on movement is minimized because the head is in midline. Objects should be positioned so that the student can look slightly down and forward. This head position will decrease the influence of abnormal reflexes (Figure 16).

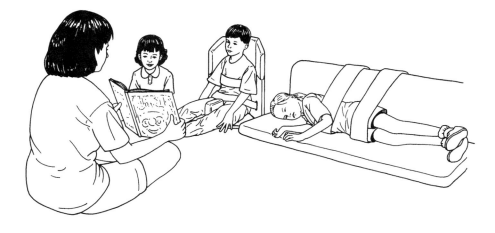

Figure 16.   These students enjoy listening to a story while being properly positioned in classroom equipment.

Wedges

Wedges come in a variety of thicknesses and lengths. The use of wedges encourages the student to raise her head and reach in prone. The symmetrical tonic neck reflex (STNR) and the tonic labyrinthine reflex (TLR) make it difficult for many students to lift their head as they lie on their stomach while supported on bent elbows. The wedge makes it easier for the student to overcome the effects of these abnormal reflexes. When positioned prone on the wedge, the student's hip flexors also receive a good stretch.

Wheelchairs

Wheelchairs are used for transport, feeding, and fine-motor and communication activities. A wide variety of models are available from several different companies. Many students with special needs require adaptations like head supports, lateral supports at the sides, and wedges between the knees to keep knees and hips in proper alignment. Special seating systems can be added to decrease the influence of abnormal tone. The COTA may not independently evaluate or prescribe a wheelchair but likely will be part of a team that gives recommendations and troubleshoots problems with seating and mobility (Ratliffe, 1998).

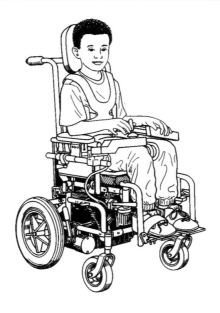

Figure 17. This power wheelchair offers independence for a non-ambulatory student.

Power wheelchairs offer non-ambulatory students the option of independent mobility (Figure 17). The COTA may train the student to use power mobility, teaching the basic skills first—proper hand position on the joystick, turning on the wheelchair, driving straight down a hallway at a safe speed, avoiding hitting other children or obstacles, and stopping prior to hitting obstacles. As the student progresses, more advanced skills are introduced, such as driving up and down curb cuts, and maneuvering on uneven ground and through classroom doorways. Classroom modifications may need to be considered to allow the student room to maneuver the power wheelchair.

Conclusion

As occupational therapy services continue to evolve, the need for COTAs no doubt will continue to grow, especially in the school-based setting. This manual attempts to provide pediatric information in a thorough and practical manner, thereby making the challenges a little bit more fun and enjoyable.

References

American Occupational Therapy Association. 1994a. *Occupational therapy roles*. Bethesda, MD: AOTA.

———. 1994b. Occupational therapy code of ethics. *American Journal of Occupational Therapy*, 48: 1037–1038.

———. 1994c. Standards of practice for occupational therapy. *American Journal of Occupational Therapy*, 48: 1039–1043.

———. 1995. Guide for supervision of occupational therapy personnel. *American Journal of Occupational Therapy*, 49: 1027–1028.

———. 1997. *Occupational therapy services for children and youth under the individuals with disabilities education act*. Bethesda, MD: AOTA.

Amundson, S.J. 1992. Handwriting: evaluation and intervention in the school setting. In *Development of hand skills in the child*. Edited by J. Case-Smith & C. Pehorski, 63–78. Rockville, MD: AOTA.

Ayres, J. 1972. *Sensory integration and learning disorders*. Los Angeles: Psychological Services.

Batshaw, M.L., & Y.M. Perret. 1992. *Children with disabilities: A medical primer*. (3rd. ed., p. 525). Baltimore: Paul H. Brookes.

Beery, K., & N. Buktenica. 1997. *Beery-Buktenica developmental test of visual-motor integration (VMI)*. New Jersey: Modern Curriculum.

Benbow, M. 1998. Activities to develop temporal & spatial awareness. Handout distributed at a workshop, August, 1998.

Berk, R.A., & G.A. DeGangi. 1983. *DeGangi-Berk test of sensory integration*. Los Angeles: Western Psychological Services.

Bissell, J., J. Fisher, C. Owens, & P. Polcyn. 1988. *Sensory motor handbook: A guide for implementing and modifying activities in the classroom*. (2d ed.) Torrance, CA: Sensory Integration International.

Bobath, K. 1966. The motor deficits in patients with cerebral palsy. *Clinics in Developmental Medicine*, 23, 191–192. Lavenham, England: Lavenham.

Bruininks, R.H. 1978. *Bruininks-Oseretsky test of motor performance.* Circle Pines, MN: American Guidance Service.

Clark, F., Z. Mailloux, & D. Parham. 1985. Sensory integration and children with learning disabilities. In *Occupational therapy for children.* Edited by P.N. Clark & A.S. Allen. St. Louis: Mosby.

Colangelo, C.A. 1993. Biomechanical frame of reference. In *Frames of reference for pediatric occupational therapy.* Edited by J. Hinojosa & P. Kramer, 233–305. Baltimore: Williams & Wilkins.

Coster, W., T. Deeney, J. Haltiwanger, & S. Haley. 1998. *School Function Assessment.* San Antonio: Therapy Skill Builders.

Curatti, T., D.D. Kahl, & C. Eldridge. 1997. *Ohio Motor Task Force Resource Guide.*

Davis, C.M., J.M. Anderson, & D. Jagger. 1979. Competency: The what, why, and how of it. *Physical Therapy*, 59, 1088–1094.

Dormans, J.P., & L. Pellegrino. 1998. *Caring for children with cerebral palsy: A team approach.* Baltimore: Paul H. Brookes.

Education for All Handicapped Children Act of 1975. U.S. Public Law 94-142. 94th Cong., 1st sess., 29 November 1975.

Eicher, P.S. 1998. Nutrition and feeding. In *Caring for children with cerebral palsy: A team approach.* Edited by J.P. Dormans & L. Pellegrino, 261–275. Baltimore: Paul H. Brookes.

Erhardt, R.P. 1989. *Erhardt developmental prehension assessment.* San Antonio: Therapy Skill Builders.

Folio, M., & R. Fewell. 1983. *Peabody developmental motor scales.* Allen, TX: DLM Teaching Resources.

Giangreco, M.F., C.J. Cloninger, & V. Iverson. 1993. *Choosing options and accommodations for children: A guide to planning inclusive education.* Baltimore: Paul H. Brookes.

Gisel, E.G. 1994. Oral motor skills following sensorimotor intervention in the moderately eating-impaired child with cerebral palsy. *Dysphagia,* 9, 180–192.

Haley, S.M., W.J. Coster, L.H. Ludlow, M.A. Haltiwanger, & P.J. Andrellos. 1992. *Pediatric evaluation of disability inventory (PEDI).* Boston: New England Medical Center Hospital and PEDI Research Group.

Hinojosa, J., P. Kramer, P. Nuse Pratt. 1996. Foundations of practice: Developmental principles, theories, and frames of reference. In *Occupational therapy for children.* Edited by J. Case-Smith, A.S. Allen, & P. Nuse Pratt, 40-44. St. Louis: Mosby.

Individuals with Disabilities Education Act (IDEA) of 1990. U.S. Public Law 101-476. (Chapter 33). 101st Cong., 2d sess., 30 October 1990.

Johnson, H., & A. Scott. 1993. *A practical approach to saliva control.* San Antonio: Communication Skill Builders.

Johnson, J. 1996. School-based occupational therapy. In *Occupational therapy for children.* Edited by J. Case-Smith, A.S. Allen, & P. Nuse Pratt, 693–716. St. Louis: Mosby.

Koomar, J. 1990. Sensory integration treatment in the public schools. In *Environment: Implications for occupational therapy practice.* Edited by S. C. Merrill, 112–141. Rockville, MD: AOTA.

McWilliam, R.A. 1995. Integration of therapy and consultative special education: A continuum in early intervention. *Infants and Young Children,* 7 (4): 29–38.

Miller, L.J. 1988. *Miller assessment for preschoolers manual.* San Antonio: The Psychological Corporation.

Minshew, N.J., & J.B. Payton. 1988. New perspectives in autism. Part I: The clinical spectrum of autism. Part II: The differential diagnosis and neurobiology of autism. *Current Problems in Pediatrics,* 18, 561–694.

Morris, S.E., & M.D. Klein. 1987. *Pre-feeding skills.* San Antonio: Therapy Skill Builders.

Parham, L., & L. Primeau. 1997. Play and occupational therapy. In *Play in occupational therapy for children.* Edited by L. Parham & L. Fazio, 2–19. St. Louis: Mosby.

Pauls, J.A., & K.L. Reed. 1996. *Quick reference to physical therapy.* Gaithersburg, MD: Aspen.

Pueschel, S.M., & F.H. Scola. 1987. Atlantoaxial: Instability in individuals with Down syndrome: Epidemiologic, radiographic and clinical studies. *Pediatrics,* 80, 555–560.

Pueschel, S.M., C. Tingey, J.E. Rynders, A.C. Crocker, & D.M. Crutcher, (Eds.). 1987. *New perspectives on Down syndrome.* Baltimore: Paul H. Brookes.

Ratliffe, K.T. 1998. *Clinical pediatric physical therapy.* St. Louis: Mosby.

Ratliffe, K.T., & W.L. Tada. 1997. Competencies for physical therapy assistant students in educational settings. Unpublished manuscript.

Reed, P. 1998. Assistive technology: Putting the puzzle together. *Disability Solutions,* 3, 3–6.

Scherzer, A.L., & I. Tscharnuter. 1982. *Early diagnosis and therapy in cerebral palsy.* New York: Marcel Dekker.

Tecklin, J.S. 1989. *Pediatric physical therapy.* Philadelphia: J.B. Lippincott.

Todd, V. 1993. Visual perceptual frame of reference: An information processing approach. In *Frames of reference for pediatric occupational therapy.* Edited by J. Hinojosa & P. Kramer, 177–232. Baltimore: Williams & Wilkins.

Usman, A., & S. Szkut. 1993. *Preschool accommodation checklist.* Watertown, MA.: Occupational Therapy Associates, P.C.

Williamson, G., M. Szczepanski, & S. Zeitlin. 1993. Coping frame of reference. In *Frames of reference for pediatric occupational therapy.* Edited by J. Hinojosa & P. Kramer, 395–435.